Basic Guide to Oral Health Education and Promotion

D0555068

Love your patients and they will do anything that you ask.
Ann Felton (1942–2007)

Ann Felton made people smile and their smiles brighter. Ann was a dental hygienist, tutor and mentor, and ran her own oral health education course for dental nurses whom she referred to as 'the darlings of dentistry'.

Ann wrote the majority of this book in difficult circumstances, yet retained her love for the subject and sense of humour throughout. This text is dedicated to Ann's life and work in making people smile.

BASIC GUIDE TO ORAL HEALTH EDUCATION AND PROMOTION

Ann Felton
RDH, Cert. Ed

Alison Chapman
RDH, FAETC

Edited by

Simon Felton
BSc (Hons), LSJ (Hons Dip)

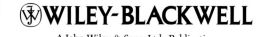WILEY-BLACKWELL

A John Wiley & Sons, Ltd., Publication

This edition first published 2009
© 2009 A. Felton, A. Chapman, & S. Felton

Blackwell Publishing was acquired by John Wiley & Sons in February 2007.
Blackwell's publishing programme has been merged with Wiley's global Scientific, Technical,
and Medical business to form Wiley-Blackwell.

Registered office
John Wiley & Sons Ltd, The Atrium, Southern Gate, Chichester, West Sussex, PO19 8SQ,
United Kingdom

Editorial offices
9600 Garsington Road, Oxford, OX4 2DQ, United Kingdom
2121 State Avenue, Ames, Iowa 50014-8300, USA

For details of our global editorial offices, for customer services and for information about how to
apply for permission to reuse the copyright material in this book please see our website at
www.wiley.com/wiley-blackwell.

Library of Congress Cataloging-in-Publication Data

Felton, Ann.
Basic guide to oral health education and promotion / Ann Felton, Alison Chapman;
edited by Simon Felton.
p. ; cm.
Includes bibliographical references and index.
ISBN 978-1-4051-6162-6 (pbk. : alk. paper)   1. Dental health education.
2. Health promotion.   I. Chapman, Alison,   II. Felton, Simon, 1970–   III. Title.
[DNLM: 1. Health Education, Dental – methods.   2. Dental Assistants.   3. Health
Promotion – methods. WU 113 F326 2009]
RK60.8.F45 2009
617.6'01 – dc22

2008039842

A catalogue record for this book is available from the British Library.

Set in 10/12.5 pt Sabon by Aptara Inc., New Delhi, India
Printed and bound in Malaysia by KHL Printing Co Sdn Bhd

1   2009

Contents

Foreword

Ann Felton and Alison Chapman have between them more than 30 years of experience in the delivery and training of oral health education. Ann designed, and has run with Alison, an exceptionally successful oral health education course in Bristol for over 10 years, with a pass rate of over 95% in the UK national examination.

This has given them great experience and understanding of the subject and the needs of students. The delivery of dental care is undergoing fundamental changes and the need to develop practice teams with skill mix makes this book very timely. Practices may well need to consider how they can make best use of their staff to help deliver oral care to their patients in the future, and oral health educators could well become an important part of this process.

This book provides a most comprehensive review of the subject. Each chapter has clearly defined learning outcomes that make it easy to read and understand. It is an ideal revision aid and basis for any member of the dental team and other health professionals wishing to know about all the aspects of oral health education. It would also be a good reference book for all practices on the subject.

Alasdair Miller
BDS, FDSRCS (Ed), DGDP, DPDS
Regional Dental Postgraduate Dean (South West)
University of Bristol

Preface

Oral health is central to our general well-being. The health of the body begins with the oral cavity, since all our daily nutrients, beneficial or otherwise, pass through it.

Knowledge in the field of oral health is changing rapidly and there is a great deal to learn. Patients need trained oral health educators (OHEs) and promoters to help prevent and control dental conditions and disease. It is vital that dental and health professionals consistently promote the same messages to avoid confusion and ultimately improve oral health within the population.

This book covers the theoretical and practical aspects of oral health education and promotion, and is the course companion for UK dental nurses studying for the NEBDN Certificate in oral health education. It is also aimed at hygienists, therapists and dentists who regularly promote and practise oral health and require up-to-date, evidence-based knowledge (including professionals and trainees in developing nations where education has proven to be a cost-effective method of improving oral health). Other professionals such as health visitors, nurses, dieticians and midwives will also find the book invaluable.

Each chapter deals with various aspects of oral health and follows the NEBDN syllabus in a logical order that will also suit other professionals who may 'dip into' relevant chapters of interest. Chapters begin with *learning outcomes*, detailing what the reader should have learnt by the end of the chapter, and conclude with self-assessment exercises. Where the word 'Remember!' appears in the text, it highlights a point particularly relevant to NEBDN students.

After reading this book, the reader should be able to:

- Confidently educate patients about diseases and conditions of the oral cavity, their treatment, management and prevention.
- Set up a preventive dental unit.
- Be aware of the wider context of oral health education and promotion in society.
- Use knowledge gained to help pass the NEBDN Certificate in oral health education.

Acknowledgements

The authors thank the following oral health education tutors for their contributions to this book:

Elizabeth Hill, RDN, Cert. OHE (NEBDN)

Frances Marriott, RDH, MRIPH, Cert Ed.

Alison Grant, RDH, FAETC

Jan Postans, RDN, Cert. OHE (NEBDN), Cert OHE (Notts.), FAETC Cert. Ed.

We are also indebted to:

Alasdair Miller, BDS, FDSRCS (Ed), DGDP, DPDS, South West Regional Postgraduate Dean, for his continued support, advice and writing the foreword;

Professor Anthony Blinkhorn, OBE, BDS, MSc, PhD, FDSRCS (Ed), FIHPE, Professor of Oral Health, University of Manchester, for support and permission to refer to his work;

Janet Goodwin, BA (Hons), RDN, Chairman NEBDN, for answering numerous questions;

Amy Brown, Managing Editor at Wiley-Blackwell, for her invaluable help and advice;

Ruth McIntosh for image design, and Dr Ian Bellamy, Dr Nick Claydon, Dr Susan Hooper, M.A.O. Lewis and Dr Nicola West for granting permission to use photography;

Elaine Tilling, MSc, RDH, DMMS, MIPHE, for permission to use some illustrations; and

Ann Dawson for her critical eye in proof checking.

Finally, Ann Felton thanks her co-author Alison Chapman for extensive research and amendments, editor son Simon without whose encouragement and hard work this book would not have been written, daughter Sarah for IT advice and husband Dave for continual patience and moral support.

SECTION 1
STRUCTURE AND FUNCTIONS OF THE ORAL CAVITY

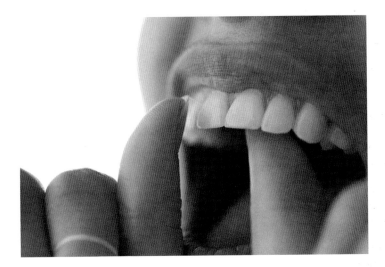

INTRODUCTION

This section comprises a revision chapter, which looks at the oral cavity in some detail. The structure of the tooth and its supporting tissues are examined, plus the eruption dates of primary and secondary dentitions.

The tongue, its functions in maintaining oral health, common conditions associated with it, and the composition and role of saliva in keeping the mouth healthy conclude the chapter.

Chapter 1

The oral cavity in health

LEARNING OUTCOMES

By the end of this chapter you should be able to:

1. Explain, in detail, the structure and function of the tissues and fluid of the oral cavity, including teeth, supporting structures, the tongue and saliva.

2. List primary and secondary dentition eruption dates.

INTRODUCTION

Before oral health educators (OHEs) can deliver dental health messages to patients, and confidently discuss oral care and disease with them, they will need a basic understanding of oral cavity anatomy (Figures 1.1 and 1.2) and how the following structures within it function:

- Teeth (including dentition)
- Periodontium (the supporting structure of the tooth)
- Tongue
- Saliva

MAIN FUNCTIONS OF THE ORAL CAVITY

The oral cavity is uniquely designed to carry out two main functions:

1. Begin the process of digestion. The cavity's hard and soft tissues, lubricated by saliva, are designed to withstand the stresses of:
   - Biting
   - Chewing
   - Swallowing
2. Produce speech.

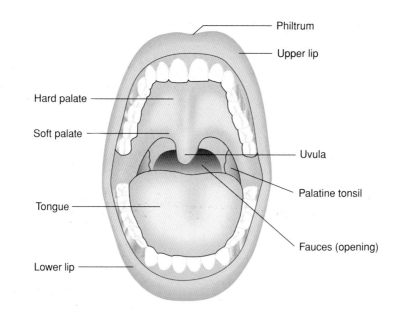

Figure 1.1 Structure of the oral cavity (© Elsevier 2002. Reproduced with permission from Reference 1)

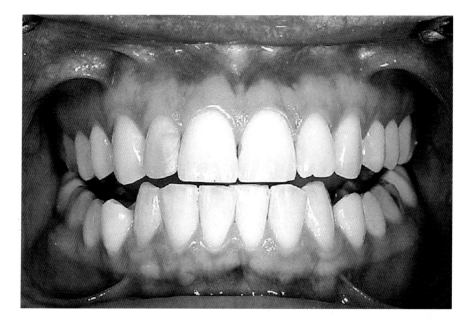

Figure 1.2 A healthy mouth (© Blackwell Publishing 2003. Reproduced with permission from Reference 2)

TEETH

Different types of teeth are designed (*shaped*) to carry out different functions. For example: canines are sharp and pointed for gripping and tearing food, while molars have flatter surfaces for chewing. Tooth form in relation to function is known as *morphology*.

Dental nurses and health care workers may remember from their elementary studies that there are two types of *dentition* (a term used to describe the *type*, *number* and *arrangement* of natural teeth).

1. Primary (*deciduous*) dentition – consisting of 20 baby teeth

2. Secondary (*permanent*) dentition – consisting of 32 adult teeth

Primary dentition

There are three types of deciduous teeth that make up the primary dentition (Figure 1.3): incisors, canines and molars (first and second). Table 1.1 details their *notation* (the code used by the dental profession to identify teeth), approximate eruption dates and functions.

Secondary dentition

There are four types of permanent teeth that make up the secondary dentition (Figure 1.4): incisors, canines, premolars and molars. Table 1.2 details their notation, approximate eruption dates and functions.

It is important to remember that these eruption dates are only approximate and vary considerably in children and adolescents. The OHE should be prepared to answer questions from parents who are worried that their child's teeth are not erupting at the same age as their friends' teeth. Parents often do not realise, for example, that no teeth fall out to make room for the first permanent molars (sixes), which appear behind the deciduous molars.

Structure of the tooth

Tooth structure (Figure 1.5, see page 10) is complex and comprises several different hard layers which protect a soft, inner pulp (nerves and blood vessels).

Organic and inorganic tooth matter

The words *organic* and *inorganic* are often mentioned in connection with tooth structure. OHEs must know what these terms mean and their percentages in hard tooth structures.

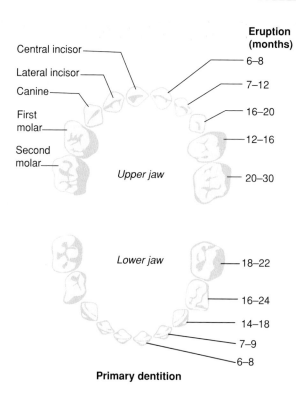

Figure 1.3 Primary dentition (© Elsevier 2002. Reproduced with permission from Reference 1)

Organic means *living* and describes the *matrix* (framework) of water, cells, fibres and proteins which make the tooth a living structure.

Inorganic means *non-living* and describes the mineral content of the tooth which gives it its strength. These minerals are complex calcium salts. (**Remember!** *calcium hydroxyapatite.*)

Table 1.3 shows the percentages of organic and inorganic matter in hard tooth structures.

Table 1.1 Primary dentition (notation, approximate eruption dates and functions)

Tooth	Notation	Approximate eruption date	Function
Incisors	(a & b)	6–12 months (usually lowers first)	Biting
First molars	(d)	12–24 months	Chewing
Canines	(c)	14–20 months	Tearing
Second molars	(e)	18–30 months	Chewing

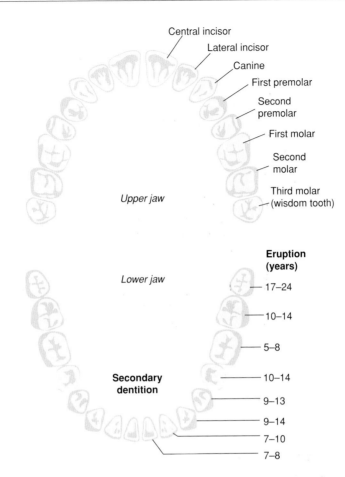

Figure 1.4 Secondary dentition (© Elsevier 2002. Reproduced with permission from Reference 1)

Table 1.2 Secondary dentition: notation, approximate eruption dates and functions

Tooth	Notation	Approximate eruption date	Function
First molars	(6)	5–8 years	Chewing
Lower central incisors	(1)	7–8 years	Biting
Upper central incisors	(1)	7–8 years	Biting
Lower lateral incisors	(2)	7–10 years	Biting
Upper lateral incisors	(2)	7–10 years	Biting
Lower canines	(3)	9–14 years	Tearing
First premolars	(4)	9–13 years	Chewing
Second premolars	(5)	10–14 years	Chewing
Upper canines	(3)	9–14 years	Tearing
Second molars	(7)	10–14 years	Chewing
Third molars	(8)	17–24 years	Chewing

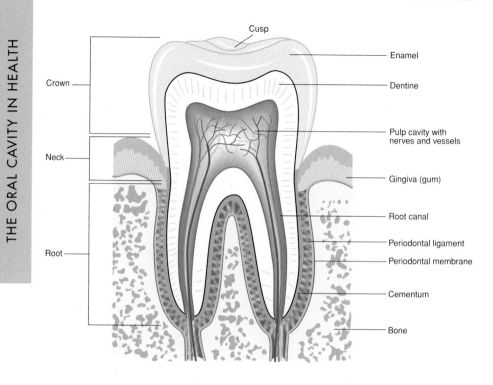

Figure 1.5 Structure of the tooth (© Elsevier 2002. Reproduced with permission from Reference 1)

It is also important that the OHE knows basic details about these three hard tooth substances, and also pulp.

Enamel

Enamel is made up of prisms (*crystals of hydroxyapatite*) arranged vertically in a wavy pattern, which give it great strength. The prisms, which resemble *fish-scales*, are supported by a matrix of organic material including keratinised (*horny*) cells and can be seen under an electronic microscope.

Table 1.3 Percentages of organic and inorganic matter in hard tooth structures

Structure	Inorganic	Organic
Enamel	96%	4%
Dentine	70%	30%
Cementum	45%	55%

Properties of enamel
Enamel is:

- The hardest substance in the human body (of similar hardness to diamond).
- Brittle – it fractures when the underlying dentine is weakened by decay (*caries*).
- Insensitive to stimuli (e.g. hot, cold and sweet substances).
- Darkens slightly with age – as secondary dentine is laid down and stains from proteins in the diet, tannin-rich food and drinks, and smoking are absorbed.

Enamel is also subject to four types of wear and tear. The OHE needs to be aware of these and be able to differentiate between them:

1. *Erosion* – usually seen on *palatal* and *lingual* (next to palate and tongue) surfaces.
2. *Abrasion* – usually seen on *cervical* (outer neck of tooth) surfaces.
3. *Attrition* – natural wear often seen on *occlusal* (biting) surfaces.
4. *Abfraction* – *notching* of the enamel close to, or beneath the *gingival margin* (gum line).

Dentine
Dentine constitutes the main bulk of the tooth and consists of millions of microscopic tubules (fine tubes), running in a curved pattern from the pulp to the enamel on the crown and the cementum on the root.

Properties of dentine
Dentine is:

- Softer than enamel, but harder than cementum and bone.
- Light yellow in colour.
- Sensitive to stimuli (e.g. hot, cold and sweet substances). Reasons for this sensitivity are not fully understood, but it usually lessens with age.
- Changes throughout life. After a tooth is fully developed, more dentine is laid down (at a slower rate than before), and is known as *secondary dentine*.

Cementum

Cementum covers the surface of the root and provides an attachment for the *periodontal ligament*. The fibres of the ligament are fixed in the cementum and in the *alveolar bone* (see supporting structures of the tooth).

Properties of cementum

Cementum is:

- Of similar hardness to bone.

- Thickens throughout life to counteract wear and tear caused by chewing and movement.

Pulp

Pulp is a soft living tissue within the pulp chamber and root canal of the tooth. It consists of blood vessels, nerves, fibres and cells. The pulp chamber shrinks with age as more secondary dentine is laid down, so that the tooth becomes less vulnerable to damage.

Supporting structures of the tooth

The *periodontium* (Figure 1.6) is the collective name for the supporting structures of the tooth. It comprises:

- Periodontal ligament

- Cementum (part of the tooth and supporting structure)

- Alveolar bone (it consists of two components: the alveolar bone proper and the alveolar process)

- Gingivae (gums)

The periodontal ligament

The periodontal ligament (*or membrane*) is a connective tissue which holds the tooth in place in the alveolar bone (assisted by cementum). The ligament is between 0.1 and 0.3 mm wide[4] and contains blood vessels, nerves, cells and *collagen fibres*.

The collagen fibres attach the tooth to the alveolar bone and run in different directions, which provide strength and flexibility and act as a *shock absorber* for the tooth; teeth need to move slightly in their sockets in order to withstand the pressures of *mastication* (chewing). Imagine what it would feel like to bite hard with teeth rigidly cemented into bone.

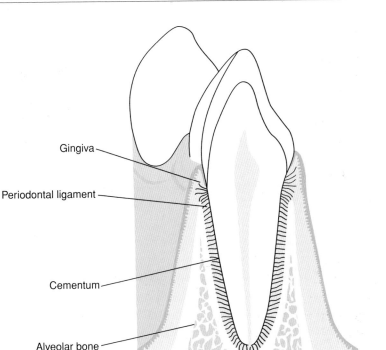

Figure 1.6 The periodontium (© Blackwell Publishing 2003. Reproduced with permission from Reference 3)

Cementum (see tooth structure, page 12)

Alveolar bone (also known as the alveolar ridge)

Alveolar bones are *horseshoe-shaped* projections of the *maxilla* (upper jaw) and *mandible* (lower jaw). They provide an attachment for the fibres of the periodontal ligament and sockets for the teeth.

Gingivae

The *gingivae* (gums) consist of pink-coloured mucous membranes and underlying fibrous tissue, covering the alveolar bone.

Gingivae are divided into four sections:

1. *Attached gingiva* (Figure 1.7) – a firm, pale pink, stippled gum tightly attached to the underlying alveolar bone. It is *keratinised (hard and firm like horn)* to withstand the friction of chewing. Its orange-peel appearance (known as *stippling*) comes from tightly packed bundles of collagen fibres that attach it to the bone. Loss of stippling is one of the signs of gingivitis.

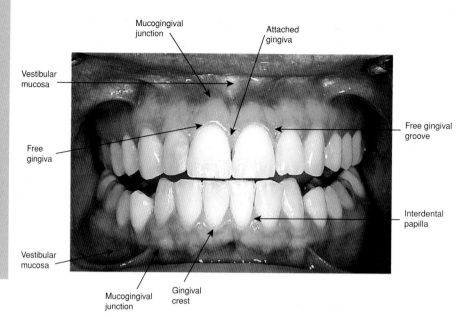

Figure 1.7 Free and attached gingiva (© Blackwell Publishing 2003. Reproduced with permission from Reference 2)

2. *Free gingiva* (Figure 1.7) – where the gum meets the tooth. It is less tightly attached and unstippled. It is also keratinised and contoured to form little points of gum between teeth – the *interdental papillae*. The indentation between attached and free gingiva is called the *free gingival groove*.

3. *Gingival crest* – the edge of the gum and interdental papillae, bordering the tooth. Behind the crest is the *gingival sulcus* (or crevice), which is not more than 2 mm in depth[4]. This base of the crevice is lined with a layer of cells called the *junctional epithelium*, which attaches the gum to the tooth. When this epithelium breaks down, in disease, periodontal ligament fibres are exposed to bacterial enzymes and toxins. As these fibres break down, a *periodontal pocket* is formed.

4. *Mucogingival junction* – the meeting point of the keratinised attached gingiva and the non-keratinised *vestibular mucosa* (soft, dark red tissue which lines the inside of lips, cheeks and the floor of the mouth).

THE TONGUE AND THE FLOOR OF THE MOUTH

The tongue is a muscular, mobile organ which lies in the floor of the mouth, and comprises four surfaces:

1. *Dorsal* (upper) surface – covered by a thick, keratinised epithelium to withstand chewing, and a large number of projections called *papillae*. These papillae contain taste buds. The dorsal surface is divided into two sections:
   - *Anterior* (front) two-thirds (against the palate)
   - *Posterior* (back) third (towards the pharynx)
2. *Ventral* (under) surface – covered by a thin mucous membrane. In the middle of the front section, the mucosa is divided into a sharp fold, which joins the tip of the tongue to the floor of the mouth (the *lingual fraenum*).
3. *Tip* – the pointed front, which can be protruded or moved around the mouth by muscular action. For a baby, the tip of the tongue is an important sensory organ, which explores and identifies objects.
4. *Root* – the deep attachment of the tongue, which forms the anterior surface of the pharynx.

Muscles of the tongue

There are two groups of tongue muscles:

1. *Intrinsic* (inside) – which can alter its shape.
2. *Extrinsic* (outside) – which move the tongue and help alter its shape.

Functions of the tongue

The main functions of the tongue are taste, mastication, *deglutition* (swallowing), speech, cleansing and protection.

Taste

The tongue (and other parts of the oral cavity) is covered with taste buds that allow us to distinguish between sweet, sour, salt and savoury tastes. An adult has approximately 9000 taste buds[4], which are mainly situated on the upper surface of the tongue (there are also some on the palate and even on the throat).

Mastication

The tongue helps to pass a soft mass of chewed food (*bolus*) along its dorsal surface and presses it against the hard palate.

Deglutition

The tongue helps pass the bolus towards the entrance of the oesophagus.

Speech

Tongue movement plays a major part in the production of different sounds.

Natural cleansing

Tongue muscles allow for tremendous movement, and the tongue can help to remove food particles from all areas of the (mouth mainly using the *tip*).

Protection

The tongue moves saliva (which has an antibacterial property) around the oral cavity.

Conditions affecting the tongue

The following conditions affect the tongue:

- *Glossitis* (inflammation of the tongue).

- Soreness of the tongue, which may be due to a variety of reasons, including anaemia, vitamin B deficiency and hormonal imbalance.

- *Black hairy tongue* – due to overgrowth of tongue papillae, stained by *chromogenic bacteria* or medication (e.g. chlorhexidine). Looks alarming, but is not serious.

- *Geographic tongue* – smooth 'maplike' irregular areas on the dorsal surface, which come and go. Harmless, but sometimes sore (often runs in families)[5].

Piercing of the tongue can also cause problems and the OHE should be able to advise patients on this matter. Tongue cleansing is also back in vogue, due to an increased awareness of halitosis[6], and tongue cleansers (e.g. TePe[®]) can help with this condition.

The floor of the mouth

The OHE need only know that the floor of the mouth consists of a muscle called the *mylohyoid* and associated structures.

SALIVA

Incredible stuff, saliva! It is often taken for granted, and patients only realise how vital it is to the well-being of the oral cavity and the whole body, when its flow is diminished.

Saliva is secreted by three major and numerous minor salivary glands. The minor glands are found in the lining of the oral cavity; on the inside of the lips, the cheeks, the palate and even the pharynx.

Major salivary glands

The three major salivary glands (Figure 1.8):

1. *Parotid gland* – situated in front of the ear. It is the largest salivary gland and produces 25% of the total volume of saliva[4]. It produces *serous* (watery) saliva, which is transported into the oral cavity by the parotid duct which opens above the upper molars. The parotid gland swells during mumps (*parotitis*).

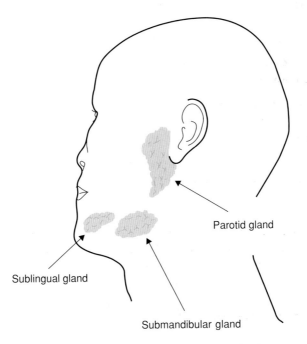

Parotid gland

Sublingual gland

Submandibular gland

Figure 1.8 Major salivary glands (© Fejerskov & Kidd. Reproduced with permission from Reference 7)

2. *Submandibular gland* – situated beneath the *mylohyoid* muscle towards the base of the mandible. It is the middle of the three glands, in both size and position, and can be said to have a 'middle role', producing a mixture of serous and mucous saliva. It produces around 70% of total saliva[4] and opens via the submandibular duct on the floor of the mouth.

   When dental nurses assist the dentist, they may occasionally notice a small 'fountain' as the saliva appears from this duct (which can also happen when yawning).

3. *Sublingual gland* – is also situated beneath the anterior floor of the mouth under the front of the tongue. It produces 5% of total saliva[4], mainly in the form of mucous which drains through numerous small ducts on the ridge of the *sublingual fold* (the section of fraenum beneath the anterior of tongue).

Composition of saliva

Saliva is made up of 99.5% water and 0.5% dissolved substances[4]. Dissolved substances include:

- Proteins – a number of different types, collectively known as *mucin*. They are also known as *glycoproteins* and provide the *substrate* (food) for plaque bacteria. They give saliva its viscosity (stickiness) and are the origin of the *salivary pellicle* (the sticky film which forms on teeth within minutes of cleaning).

- Enzymes – there are many but the OHE need only remember the main ones: *salivary amylase (ptyalin)* and *lysozyme*.

- *Serum proteins* – *albumin* and *globulin* (saliva is formed from *serum*, the watery basis of blood).

- Waste products – urea and uric acid.

- Gases – oxygen, nitrogen and carbon dioxide in solution. The latter vaporises when it enters the mouth and is given off as a gas.

- Inorganic ions – including sodium, sulphate, potassium, calcium, phosphate and chloride. The important ones to remember are calcium and phosphate ions which are concerned with *remineralisation* of the teeth after an acid attack and the development of calculus.

Functions of saliva

There are eight main functions of saliva:

1. Mastication and deglutition – mucous helps to form the food bolus.

2. Oral hygiene – washing and antibacterial action helps to control disease of the oral cavity. Lysozyme controls bacterial growth. This is why saliva is said to have antibacterial properties and why animals (and humans!) instinctively lick their wounds.

3. Speech – a lubricant. For example: nervousness = production of adrenaline = reduction in saliva = dry mouth.

4. Taste – saliva dissolves substances and allows the taste buds to recognise taste.

5. Helps maintain water balance (of body) – when water balance is low, saliva is reduced, producing thirst.

6. Excretion – trace amounts of urea and uric acid (a minor role in total body excretion).

7. Digestion – salivary amylase begins the breakdown of cooked starch. A relatively minor role in the whole digestive process but important in relation to sucrose intake and oral disease.

8. Buffering action – helps to maintain the neutral pH of the mouth. The bicarbonate ion is vital to the health of the mouth as it is concerned with the buffering action of saliva. The resting pH of the mouth (when no food has just been consumed) is around 6.8. This is neutral (i.e. neither acid nor alkaline). (pH is a symbol used to indicate measurement of acidity or alkalinity of substances or liquids, and stands for the German term *potenz Hydrogen*.)

Facts about saliva

Here are some general points of interest about saliva:

- Composition varies with individuals.
- More is secreted when required (reflex action).
- Composition varies according to what is being eaten (e.g. more mucous with meat).
- Average amount produced daily by adults is 0.5–1 litre. Certain medical conditions and disabilities result in the overproduction of saliva, resulting in

dribbling (e.g. patients with Down's syndrome and Parkinson's disease, and fungal infections such as *angular cheilitis*).

- Flow almost ceases during sleep.
- Saliva is sterile until it enters the mouth.
- Salivary tests can be used to solve crimes, since saliva contains *deoxyribonucleic acid* (DNA) which can be used to help identify individuals. Dental companies sell salivary testing kits, which can be used by OHEs to demonstrate salivary pH to patients.

Other additives within the mouth

Although saliva entering the mouth is sterile, it soon loses this property as it collects organic material already present, including:

- Microorganisms: bacteria (mainly *streptococci*), viruses (e.g. *herpes simplex*) and fungi (e.g. *candida albicans*).
- *Leucocytes* (*neutrophils* or specialised white blood cells) which fight infection. Not present in *edentulous* (toothless) babies or in saliva collected from the duct, so presumed to come from gingival crevice after teeth erupt.
- Dietary substances (meal remains). Amounts of dissolved substances vary between and within individuals.

SELF-ASSESSMENT

1. Draw a diagram of a tooth in its socket, labelling enamel, dentine, cementum, pulp, the periodontal ligament, alveolar bone and gingivae.
2. Briefly explain the meaning of *organic* and *inorganic*.
3. How does dentine change with age? What effect does this change have upon:
   - The pulp chamber
   - Sensitivity
4. How does cementum respond to wear and tear on the tooth?
5. What does pulp consist of?
6. Write a brief description of the tongue, and list its functions.
7. What is the name for the structure which makes up the floor of the mouth?
8. Draw a diagram to show the position of the major salivary glands, and list five functions of saliva.

9. List the supporting structures of the tooth, and the collective name for these structures.

10. List the approximate eruption dates of primary and secondary teeth.

REFERENCES

1. Thibodeau, G.A., Patton, K.T. (2002) *Anatomy and Physiology*, 5th edn. Mosby, Missouri, USA.
2. Lang, N.P., Mobelli, A., Attström, R. (2003) *Dental Plaque and Calculus*. In Lindhe, J., Karring, T., Lang, N.P. (Eds): *Clinical Periodontology and Implant Dentistry*, 4th edn, pp. 81–105. Blackwell Munksgaard, Oxford.
3. Lindhe, J., Karring, T., Araújo, M. (2003) *Anatomy of the Periodontium*. In Lindhe, J., Karring, T., Lang, N.P. (Eds): *Clinical Periodontology and Implant Dentistry*, 4th edn, pp. 3–49. Blackwell Munksgaard, Oxford.
4. Collins, W.J., Walsh, T., Figures, K. (1999) *A Handbook for Dental Hygienists*, 4th edn. Butterworth Heinemann, Oxford.
5. Cawson, R.A. (1981) *Aids to Oral Pathology and Diagnosis*, Churchill Livingstone (Medial Division of Longman Group), Edinburgh.
6. Tilling, E. (2007) *Xerostomia, Your Patients and You*. Lecture given at Gloucester Independent Hygienists' Study Day, Berkley, Gloucestershire, 16 March 2007.
7. Fejerskov, O., Kidd, E. (Eds) (2003) *Dental Caries: The Disease and its Clinical Management*. Blackwell Munksgaard, Oxford.

SECTION 2
DISEASES AND CONDITIONS OF THE ORAL CAVITY

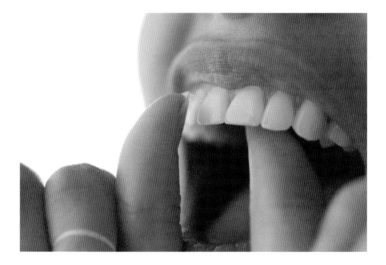

This section explores the reasons for, and the effects of, the breakdown of oral health, and details advice that should be given to patients to prevent disease and restore a good standard of oral health.

What causes dental disease?

There is, of course, no brief answer. The determinants are many and complex, and more often than not a combination of factors are involved in the development of a particular condition or disease: cultural, environmental, socioeconomic, diet and lifestyle (the latter has much to answer for). Education in these areas is thus vital in controlling dental disease.

Chapter 2
Plaque, calculus and staining

LEARNING OUTCOMES

By the end of this chapter you should be able to:

1. List the main bacteria involved in the development and maturation of plaque.
2. Distinguish between *aerobic* and *anaerobic* bacteria and their effects on oral tissues.
3. List secondary factors in the development of plaque.
4. Explain the causes, effects and treatment of calculus and tooth staining.

INTRODUCTION

Oral health educators (OHEs) need an understanding of plaque and calculus, and their roles in the development of common dental diseases such as caries, gingivitis and periodontitis.

PLAQUE

Most people have heard of *plaque*, but few would be able to explain its composition.

Plaque is a substance containing bacteria and debris, which collects on the surfaces of teeth (Figure 2.1). Even in people with good toothbrushing skills, one would need to brush and floss approximately every 3 min in order to prevent plaque from forming (M. Midda, personal communications).

Where is plaque found?

The most common sites where plaque is found are occlusal pits and fissures, cervical margins of the teeth, and in *periodontal pockets*.

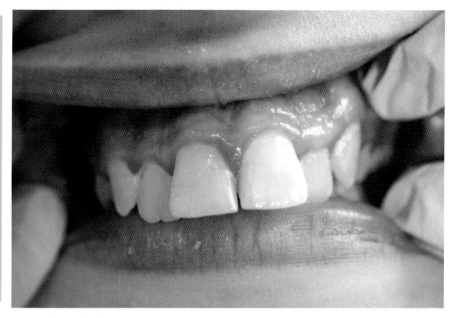

Figure 2.1 Plaque (© Carole Hollins. Reproduced with permission from Reference 1)

Formation of plaque

Saliva plays a large part in the formation of plaque. It is a complex fluid and contains many nutrients of blood, which continually coat a transparent film of *glycoproteins* (complex sugars and proteins) over the teeth. This *film* is known as the *salivary pellicle*, and the mucous it contains makes it sticky and difficult to remove.

Within a few hours after brushing the salivary pellicle is colonised by millions of microorganisms (both 'good and bad'), which feed on sugars and starches present, although plaque bacteria can multiply to a lesser degree without this substrate. At any given time, there are around 300 species and several hundred billion microorganisms in the oral cavity[2].

In a healthy mouth the 'good guys' kill off the 'baddies', but when illness or antibiotics (for example) upsets the balance of the mouth's *flora*, or when teeth are not cleaned often and/or appropriately, the villains can get the upper hand. Bacteria are the first microorganisms to colonise the salivary pellicle, and form a large colony within 3 h following toothbrushing. This colonised salivary pellicle constitutes *early plaque*.

Classification of bacteria

Bacteria are classified by whether they need oxygen or not to survive and the colour that they stain in laboratory tests (known as *Gram's staining*).

Aerobic bacteria

The majority of bacteria in a healthy mouth come from the oxygen-dependent (*aerobic*) *streptococci group* which colonise areas of the mouth where oxygen is readily available. When resistance is lowered they can give rise to sore throats and other illnesses, but are less harmful than their non-oxygen-dependent (*anaerobic*) relatives[4].

Aerobic bacteria are also known as *gram-positive* bacteria (staining blue/purple after the application of dye).

The most common species of streptococci (*Sing. Streptococcus*) bacteria found in the oral cavity are:

- *Streptococcus sanguis*
- *Streptococcus mutans*
- *Streptococcus mitis*
- *Streptococcus salivarius*

Aerobic bacteria feed on sucrose from the human diet, and in doing so, produce sticky substances that enable other more harmful organisms to attach themselves, causing plaque to become more dense and harmful to tissues within hours.

Anaerobic bacteria

The more *pathogenic* (disease causing) bacteria do not need oxygen to survive and can hide in areas of the mouth such as periodontal pockets, which render them difficult to remove. They are also often known as *gram-negative* bacteria (staining red/pink after the application of dye).

Examples of gram-negative bacteria are:

- *Fusiforms*
- *Vibrios*
- *Spirochaetes* – these have the unique ability to invade tissues

Maturation of plaque

Poor plaque removal is the primary cause of mature plaque. When plaque is left on teeth (often when they are cleaned ineffectively), it begins to *mature* – bacteria numbers increase and more harmful microorganisms appear – and it becomes increasingly harmful to both hard and soft tissues.

PLAQUE, CALCULUS AND STAINING

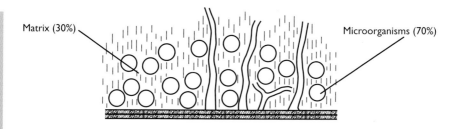

Figure 2.2 Mature plaque (© Ruth McIntosh. Reproduced with permission)

Mature plaque (Figure 2.2) consists of:

- 70% microorganisms (anaerobic bacteria, fungi, viruses)
- 30% matrix (the framework that holds it together)

Microorganisms

After 24 h without brushing, a clinically detectable layer of plaque is formed. As this matures, gram-negative bacteria vastly increase in numbers, organising themselves into colonies. These colonies make up the *biofilm*, which has been likened to communities within cities[4]. The inhabitants share resources and repel 'invaders', which individually they would be unable to do. If this plaque is not removed after 7–10 days, microorganisms present will include aerobic and anaerobic bacteria, viruses and fungi.

Anaerobic bacteria
Anaerobic bacteria produce enzymes and toxins. These potentially harmful substances can cause *gingivitis* and subsequently periodontitis.

Fungi
Fungi such as *Candida albicans* (oral thrush) are commonly found in plaque. As with bacteria, these do not affect oral health unless the body's resistance is lowered and the immune system is upset.

Viruses
The most common virus in the oral cavity is *herpes simplex*, which gives rise to cold sores.

The matrix

As well as providing an abundant food source for bacteria, the salivary pellicle also collects any other debris present in the mouth which forms the *matrix* (in which the colonising bacteria feed and reproduce).

The following substances make up the matrix:

- Proteins and carbohydrates (from food debris)
- Dead cells (from oral tissues)
- Red blood cells
- White blood cells
- Enzymes and toxins (produced by bacteria)
- Lactic acid
- *Antigens* (involved in an immune response)

Secondary factors in the retention of plaque

The importance of the following secondary factors in the retention of plaque (and therefore in the development of dental disease) should not be under-estimated:

- Large or uneven restorations
- Bridges
- Crowns with poor margins
- Implants
- Dentures
- Orthodontic appliances
- Pockets

Plaque control

The following measures should be taken to prevent the build-up of plaque:

- Physical (i.e. toothbrushing and flossing)
- Chemical (e.g. *chlorhexidine mouthwashes*) – not needed by all patients
- A low sucrose diet

Remember! The enzymes and toxins of anaerobic bacteria in mature plaque are the primary causes of *gingivitis* and *periodontitis*.

PLAQUE, CALCULUS AND STAINING

CALCULUS

Calculus is the mineralised or calcified bacterial plaque deposit that forms on teeth and other solid structures in the mouth. It plays a role in the development of periodontal disease by attracting more plaque.

Patients sometimes refer to calculus (a Latin word meaning *stone*) as *tartar* or *scale*. When talking to patients, it is worth mentioning that these three terms mean the same thing. Patients often know what calculus looks like and complain of its build-up around the lower incisors.

Calculus consists of:

- 70% inorganic salts

- 30% microorganisms and organic material

There are two main types of calculus – *supragingival* which forms above the gingival margin, and *subgingival* which forms in the periodontal pocket.

Supragingival calculus

Supragingival calculus (Figure 2.3) begins to form after 2–14 days of inadequate plaque removal[5], depending upon the individual's cleaning ability and mineral

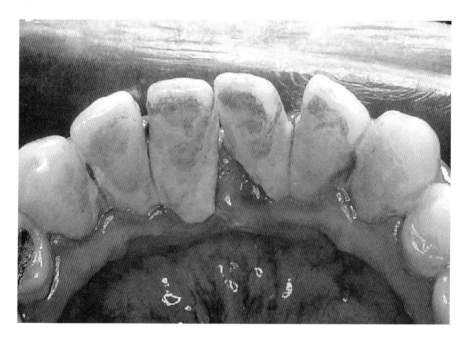

Figure 2.3 Abundance of supragingival calculus deposits and inflammation (© Blackwell Publishing 2003. Reproduced with permission from Reference 3)

content of their saliva. Most supragingival calculus is found around the salivary ducts, i.e. behind the lower central incisors and on the *buccal* (cheek) surfaces of the upper first and second molars.

It is always preceded by plaque accumulation that becomes hardened (*calcified*) by the mineral salts in saliva (i.e. calcium and phosphate salts become incorporated into sticky plaque causing calcification).

Some patients have more supragingival calculus than others, and this is because:

- They have relatively more calcium phosphate ions in saliva, and/or

- They do not remove plaque effectively, and so there is material present for saliva to calcify.

Patients cannot remove calculus with a brush or floss once it has hardened, and because it has a rough texture more plaque adheres and the process of *calcification* begins again. Dentists and hygienists scale and polish teeth to remove supragingival calculus (and help prevent periodontal disease).

Subgingival calculus

Subgingival calculus (Figure 2.4) is less obvious to the patient and is found below the gum margin in periodontal pockets. It is often black in colour and is

PLAQUE, CALCULUS AND STAINING

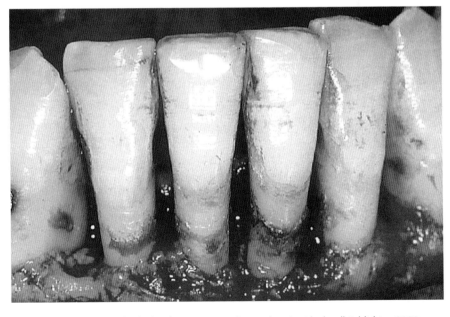

Figure 2.4 Sub-gingival calculus during a surgical procedure (© Blackwell Publishing 2003. Reproduced with permission from Reference 3)

formed when minerals from fluid in the gingival crevice (*crevicular fluid*) come into contact with plaque. (The dark colour is derived from the breakdown of blood constituents resulting from *ulceration* in the crevice).

Subgingival calculus is often hard and difficult to remove. Its presence is much more significant than supragingival deposits as it indicates that gingivitis has progressed to periodontitis.

STAINING

Dental staining describes a pigmented deposit on the surface of a tooth or teeth. There are two types of tooth staining – *intrinsic* and *extrinsic*.

Intrinsic staining

Intrinsic staining occurs within the tooth structure during its development (i.e. before birth, or during early childhood), and before it erupts (except in cases of *pulpal death*, usually caused by trauma). Intrinsic stains cannot be removed, although tooth whitening can conceal them. The whitened tooth will continue to darken with age, but the whitening process can be 'topped up' so that intrinsic stains are still concealed. Causes of intrinsic staining include:

- *Tetracycline* (an antibiotic). Taken by a small child or passed to the foetus when the mother is pregnant (it is now illegal in the UK to prescribe this drug to pregnant women, or children under 12 years old).

- Fluoride taken in excess (tablets and/or swallowing toothpaste), or naturally occurring high levels in water supply. This is called *fluorosis*.

- *Systemic* (body system) upset. Acute illness of a small child or pregnant mother can cause *hypoplasia* (the underdevelopment of a tooth and therefore enamel).

- Rare, inherited imperfections in enamel or dentine.

- Death of pulp. This causes the tooth to progressively darken.

Extrinsic staining

Extrinsic staining occurs on enamel surfaces after a tooth has erupted, when pigments from the following substances stain the salivary pellicle:

- Tannin (in tea, coffee and red wine)
- Tobacco

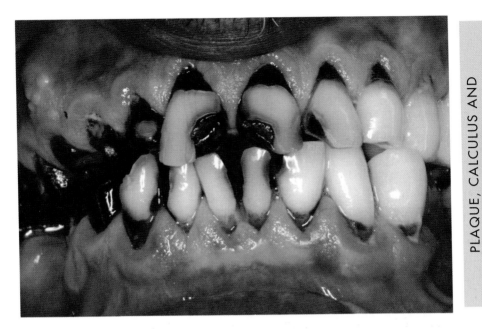

Figure 2.5 Extrinsic staining caused by betel nut chewing (© Dr Susan Hooper, Bristol University. Reproduced with permission)

- Betel nut (*paan*) chewing in certain ethnic groups (Figure 2.5)
- Chlorhexidine (present in chlorhexidine gluconate mouthwashes)
- Iron supplements

Extrinsic stains are usually removed fairly easily by scaling and polishing.

Occasionally, patients with clean mouths develop a dark stain on lingual and palatal tooth surfaces which is difficult to remove. This is called *black stain* and the cause is unknown. Children may also develop *green stain*, when the membrane covering an erupting tooth remains and is stained by bacteria. This is usually seen on the buccal surfaces of the upper incisors, can look unsightly and is often difficult to remove.

SELF-ASSESSMENT

1. Briefly explain the development and maturation of plaque, mentioning the bacteria involved.

2. Explain the difference between aerobic and anaerobic bacteria, and their effects upon oral tissues.

3. List the secondary factors in the development of plaque.

PLAQUE, CALCULUS AND STAINING

4. How does supragingival calculus form and where is it found?

5. How does subgingival calculus form, where is it found and why is it black?

6. What is the role of calculus in the development of periodontal disease, and how is it treated?

7. Define intrinsic and extrinsic staining.

8. List the factors that can cause intrinsic staining.

9. List the substances that can cause extrinsic staining.

10. How can staining be removed or improved by the dental professional?

REFERENCES

1. Hollins, C. (2008) *Basic Guide to Dental Procedures*. Wiley Blackwell, Oxford.
2. Alavi, A. (2000) *The Colgate Lecture*, BDHA General Assembly of Members, Royal Commonwealth Society, London, 2 December 2000.
3. Lang, N.P., Mobelli, A., Attström, R. (2003) *Dental Plaque and Calculus*. In Lindhe, J., Karring, T., Lang, N.P. (Eds): *Clinical Periodontology and Implant Dentistry*, 4th edn, pp. 81–105. Blackwell Munksgaard, Oxford.
4. Lindhe, J., Karring, T., Lang, N. (2003) *Clinical Periodontology and Implant Dentistry*, 4th edn. Blackwell Munksgaard, Oxford.
5. Collins, W.J., Walsh, T., Figures, K. (1999) *A Handbook for Dental Hygienists*, 4th edn. Butterworth Heinemann, Oxford.

Chapter 3
Chronic gingivitis

LEARNING OUTCOMES

By the end of this chapter you should be able to:

1. Define *inflammation* and *chronic gingivitis*, and describe the primary and secondary causes of chronic gingivitis.
2. Explain the difference between *signs* and *symptoms*, and list the signs and symptoms of chronic gingivitis.
3. Explain how to treat chronic gingivitis.

WHAT IS CHRONIC GINGIVITIS?

Chronic gingivitis is the persistent inflammation of the gums (Figures 3.1 and 3.2). (When a word ends in 'itis' it usually describes an inflammatory condition of a body tissue. For example: tonsill*itis* is inflammation of the tonsils.)

Chronic gingivitis is the condition that the oral health educator (OHE) will probably encounter most frequently. It is thought to affect at least 40% of the world's population, and can be present in children[1].

Since, initially, it rarely causes pain and affected gums can appear relatively normal, many sufferers are unaware that anything is wrong and will tell the educator that their gums have bled when brushing for years. OHEs will often hear comments such as: 'I thought it was normal for my gums to bleed', or 'My gums always bleed when I have a new toothbrush'.

One of the roles of the OHE is to dispel these myths and promote the message that 'healthy gums do not bleed'. In order to do this, the educator needs to understand gingivitis and its causes, and have a basic knowledge of the body's inflammatory process.

Primary cause of chronic gingivitis

The primary cause of chronic gingivitis is poor oral hygiene, leading to irritation from the enzymes and toxins of anaerobic bacteria in mature plaque.

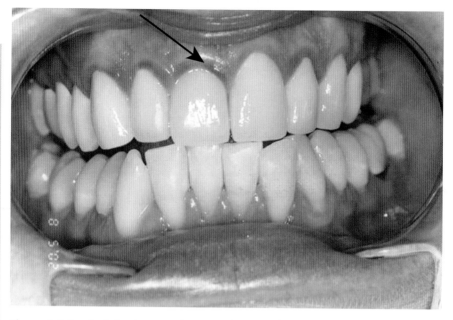

Figure 3.1 Localised chronic marginal gingivitis (© Dr Nicola West, Bristol University. Reproduced with permission)

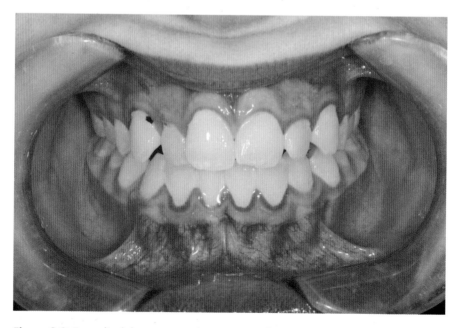

Figure 3.2 Generalised chronic marginal gingivitis (© Alison Chapman. Reproduced with permission)

Secondary causes of chronic gingivitis

Secondary causes include:

- Plaque retention, due to:
  - Overhanging fillings.
  - Ill-fitting crowns, bridges and dentures.
  - Implants.
  - Orthodontic appliances.
  - Calculus.
- Hormone changes during:
  - Pregnancy.
  - Puberty.
  - Menopause.
- Drug-induced:
  - Beta blockers (for high blood pressure) can cause *gingival overgrowth* (overgrowth of tissue).
  - *Phenytoin* (a drug used for epilepsy) – gingival overgrowth results in plaque retention and gingivitis.
- *Lip apart posture* (formerly called *mouth breathing*). The dryness of the attached gingivae in people whose lips are naturally parted when relaxed, increases the likelihood of plaque retention and *labial gingivitis*.

Inflammation

The OHE needs a basic knowledge of the body's inflammatory process in order to explain gingivitis to patients who need to deal with the condition.

Inflammation is the process by which the body defends itself against attack from:

- Physical sources (e.g. a blow to the mouth or a scratch from a toothbrush bristle).
- Chemical sources (e.g. an aspirin burn or a reaction to chemicals used in dentistry).
- Microorganisms (e.g. invasion by bacteria, viruses or fungi).

Stages of inflammation

Remember! The four stages of inflammation are also features of chronic gingivitis:

1. Redness (*rubor*).

2. Swelling (*tumor*).

3. Heat (*calor*).

4. Pain (*dolor*) – rare in chronic gingivitis, though patients sometimes complain of sore gums.

The words in brackets are Latin and they may help in remembering these stages by association (ruby from *rubor*, tumour from *tumor*, calories from *calor* and doleful from *dolor*).

Other signs and symptoms of chronic gingivitis

Signs are what the dental professional notices on examination; *symptoms* are what the patient may complain of. Signs and symptoms of chronic gingivitis are reversible and will disappear if inflammation is resolved by improved oral hygiene.

Signs

The dental professional may notice:

- Loss of *stippling* – the *orange peel* effect seen in healthy, attached gingivae, caused by bundles of collagen fibres beneath the epithelium. These bundles are damaged by the inflammatory process and stippling disappears.

- False pocketing – caused by swelling of the marginal gingivae. There is no breach of the junctional epithelium so the periodontal ligament remains intact.

- Loss of contour – the gingivae lose their pointed shape, due to swelling.

- Loss of consistency – gingivae lose their firmness and become soft and spongy.

Symptoms

The patient may complain of:

- Bleeding on brushing – this is often the first thing that patients notice. They may also mention that their gums bleed when eating crisp foods such as apples, or they may find blood on their pillow in the morning.

- Halitosis (*fetor oris*) – 'My breath smells'. May be caused by bleeding, but more likely to be noticed in chronic periodontitis when debris becomes trapped in pockets.

- Pain (rarely) – usually from trauma of vigorous brushing with a stiff brush, or when another condition, such as the hormonal changes during pregnancy, is present.

Remember! *Signs* are what the professional notices; *symptoms* are what the patient complains of.

Treatment of chronic gingivitis

Treatment should include:

- Oral hygiene instruction, encouragement and motivation.

- Removal of plaque retentive sites.

- Chemical (chlorhexidine mouthwash).

- Regular monitoring, including scaling, polishing and reinforcement of oral health instruction (OHI).

SELF-ASSESSMENT

1. Run your nails or a blunt object such as a ruler along your forearm and observe the reaction. What did you notice first? What did you notice immediately afterwards? You should have noticed that:

   - The scratch marks appeared white. You are observing the body's instant reaction to protect. The rate of blood flow in the tiny vessels beneath the skin slows as they constrict, and *neutrophils* (white blood cells which defend the body against attack) escape into the tissues to begin the defence mechanism.
   - The scratch marks turned red. This is caused by the blood vessels dilating to allow an increase in blood volume (and white blood cells) to the area, and shows that the *inflammatory process* has begun. The body is preparing to repair the damage. The continued redness is because the irritant has not been removed.

   The same mechanism occurs in gingivae when they are attacked by the enzymes and toxins of mature plaque. Clinicians will notice the redness of early gingivitis. Patients will probably not notice anything until it has been present for a while and their gums begin to bleed.

2. List the four stages of inflammation (including their Latin names if it helps).

3. Define *signs*, and list four signs that the dental professional may observe in a patient with chronic gingivitis.

4. Define *symptoms*, and pretend you are a patient explaining your gingivitis symptoms to the dentist. Write a short paragraph, describing how you are affected.

5. What is the primary cause of chronic gingivitis?

6. List four factors that encourage the retention of plaque.

7. List four secondary causes of chronic gingivitis.

8. List the treatments for chronic gingivitis.

REFERENCE

1. Collins, W.J., Walsh, T., Figures, K. (1999) *A Handbook for Dental Hygienists*, 4th edn. Butterworth Heinemann, Oxford.

Chapter 4
Chronic periodontitis

WHAT IS CHRONIC PERIODONTITIS?

Chronic periodontitis is the inflammation and gradual destruction of the periodontium (the supporting structure of the tooth).

Primary causes of chronic periodontitis

'Periodontal diseases arise from a complex interaction between microbial factors and a susceptible host[1].'

Chronic periodontitis is often, but not always, a progression of chronic gingivitis, and is primarily caused by the enzymes and toxins of mature plaque bacteria which gradually break down the tissues of the periodontium[1]. However, such damage does not always progress to periodontitis and research continues into its *aetiology* (causes), which are now regarded as more complex than previously thought.

Remember! It is important that OHEs can distinguish between *chronic gingivitis* (the continual but superficial inflammation of the gingivae) and *chronic periodontitis*.

Secondary factors in the development of periodontitis

Secondary factors are important in the development of periodontitis, and include:

- Poor oral hygiene – failure to clean interdentally leading to plaque accumulation in pockets.

- Smoking – has now been shown to be a major contributing factor and can prevent the control of bone loss in an otherwise clean mouth. Over 50% of patients under 33 years old who have periodontal disease are smokers, and 90% of patients with advanced periodontal disease are smokers[1].

- Plaque-retention factors – poorly finished/worn fillings, dentures, crowns, bridges and supra- and subgingival calculus.

- Crowding and malocclusion – one of the reasons for carrying out orthodontic treatment in childhood is to prevent periodontal disease from occurring later. Bone loss associated with malocclusion, caused by abfraction, is usually localized and not associated with poor oral hygiene.

- Carious cavities – plaque retentive ledges.

- High *fraenal insertion* – usually found buccally on lower anteriors. The *fraenum* is a fold of mucous membrane which limits the movement of the lower lip. If the insertion of the membrane is high on the gingiva, it can cause plaque accumulation and gingival recession.

- Medically compromised patients – patients with diabetes, kidney dialysis and immunological disorders are more likely to develop chronic periodontitis, because their immune system has been compromised.

Who does it affect?

Chronic periodontitis (Figure 4.1) is thought to affect around 95% of the world's adults[2] at some stage in life. The severity of the disease varies and there are other factors involved, which influence the degree to which individuals are affected. Probably only 10–15% of sufferers will lose teeth as a result.

Recent research[1] links untreated periodontal disease to spontaneous miscarriage, premature births and low birth-weights (though unsubstantiated). The disease is also thought to be a higher risk factor than high blood pressure/high cholesterol in causing certain heart diseases; it has recently been shown that

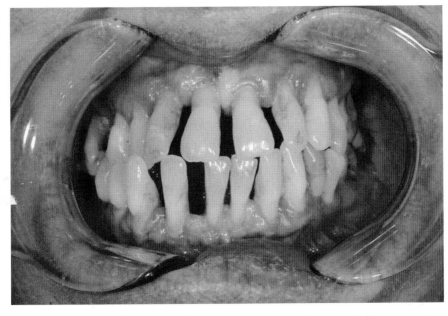

Figure 4.1 Chronic adult periodontal disease (© Dr Ian Bellamy. Reproduced with permission)

bacteria involved in the development of periodontal disease can invade and infect human arterial cells[3].

Features of chronic periodontitis

Features include:

- Often occurs in middle age.

- Usually progresses slowly.

- Can have unpredictable bursts of activity (active phases may need clinical intervention).

- Can result from the progression of gingivitis, but not always – many people have gingivitis for years but do not develop periodontitis. This is due to a factor called the *host response*, which takes into account other factors, such as a patient's general health, immune system, smoking and inherited traits.

- Patients can present with no obvious visual clinical signs (in some cases the tissues can look quite healthy). Only pocket probing and radiographs will identify the loss of supporting structures. Dental professionals in the UK have a *duty of care* to diagnose the disease in its early stages.

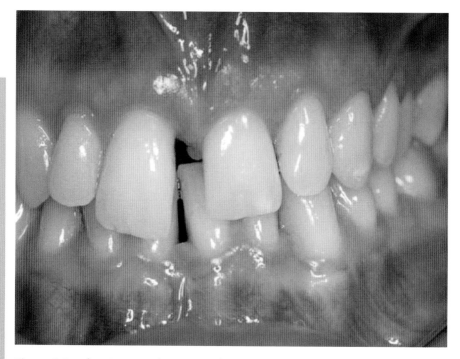

Figure 4.2 Drifting (© Dr Nicola West, Bristol University. Reproduced with permission)

Signs of chronic periodontitis

In the early stages of the disease the dental professional will notice:

- A variable degree of chronic gingivitis. Some patients still have chronic gingivitis, others not.
- Bleeding on deep probing.
- The presence of subgingival calculus.
- Gingival recession.
- Bone loss – may be horizontal or vertical (and only apparent on X-rays).

In the advanced stage of the disease the dental professional will notice:

- Periodontal abscess (invasion of pocket organisms into surrounding tissues).
- Drifting and/or mobility of teeth – due to loss of attachment (Figure 4.2). Forty-three per cent UK adults over 16 years old have more than 4 mm attachment loss and 8% more than 6 mm[4].

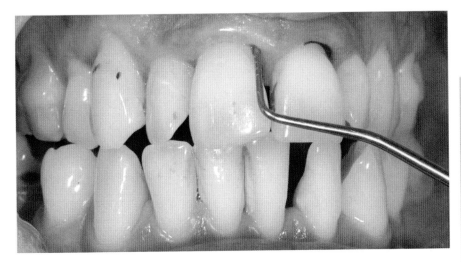

Figure 4.3 True pocketing (© Dr Nicola West, Bristol University. Reproduced with permission)

- Loss of attachment, characterised by true pocketing (Figure 4.3), which may be either:

  - *Suprabony* – when the base of the pocket is above the alveolar bone crest.

  - *Infrabony* – when the base of the pocket is below the crest of alveolar bone.

Symptoms of chronic periodontitis

In the early stages of periodontitis the patient may complain of:

- Recession – gums recede and teeth may be *hot* and *cold* sensitive.
- Halitosis or a *bad taste* due to accumulation of bacteria in pockets and pus formation.

In the advanced stage of periodontitis the patient may complain of:

- Drifting – teeth begin to move
- Mobility – often just one or two loose teeth initially
- Pain (sometimes – from periodontal abscess)
- Pus oozing from pockets

CHRONIC PERIODONTITIS

Treatment and management

Treatment and management of chronic periodontitis includes the following:

- Encouragement and help to stop smoking.
- Regular maintenance and monitoring by:

  - Patient – effective regular plaque removal using manual or powered brush, and either floss, tape, interdental brushes or wood sticks, plus chlorhexidine mouthwash.

  - Dentist – pocket charting, bleeding indices and removal of plaque retentive factors.

  - Hygienist – scaling, root surface debridement and chemical treatment (e.g. chlorhexidine impregnated chip placed in pocket).

- Antibiotics – systemic or local (if dentist feels necessary).
- Surgery – removal of pockets and re-contouring of gingivae.

SELF-ASSESSMENT

1. Define chronic periodontitis.
2. What are the primary causes of chronic periodontitis? (Mention three factors.)
3. List the secondary factors in its development.
4. What is the main distinguishing feature between chronic periodontitis and chronic gingivitis?
5. How would the dental professional diagnose early chronic periodontitis? (Mention three signs.)
6. List four signs that the dental professional may notice when the disease has progressed.
7. What might the patient with early periodontitis complain of?
8. What might the patient notice as the disease progresses?
9. Describe how the patient, dentist and hygienist should each manage and treat the disease.

REFERENCES

1. Galgut, P. (2006) *Current Concepts in Periodontology*. Paper given at Gloucester Independent Dental Hygienists' Practical Periodontics Meeting, Cheltenham, Gloucestershire, 1 December 2006.
2. Griffiths, J., Boyle, S. (1993) *Colour Guide to Holistic Oral Care, a Practical Approach*, 4th edn. Mosby-Year Book Europe, London.
3. British Dental Hygienists' Association (August 2006) *DH Contact*, The Newsletter of the British Dental Hygienists' Association, BDHA, London.
4. Office for National Statistics (2000) *Adult Dental Health Survey (1998): Oral Health in the United Kingdom, 1998*, Stationery Office Books, London.

CHRONIC PERIODONTITIS

Chapter 5

Other common oral diseases and conditions

LEARNING OUTCOMES

By the end of this chapter you should be able to:

1. List conditions and diseases which affect the oral cavity.

2. Write brief notes on *flash cards*, summarising the main features and management of these conditions and diseases (a revision exercise for UK dental nurses taking the NEBDN exam).

INTRODUCTION

Many conditions and diseases affect the oral cavity; indeed, certain systemic conditions such as diabetes and *lichen planus* are diagnosed through the oral cavity. This chapter explores the more common conditions and diseases that the oral health educator (OHE) is likely to encounter.

PERIODONTAL ABSCESS

A periodontal abscess (Figure 5.1) is a localised collection of pus, also sometimes referred to as a *lateral periodontal abscess*, as it occurs on the side of the root or in the *furcation* (the division between two roots). It is usually, although not always, a development of advanced periodontitis.

Aetiology (*cause*)

A periodontal abscess usually develops from a periodontal pocket – as organisms invade tissues and the outlet is blocked by a foreign body or food debris. It

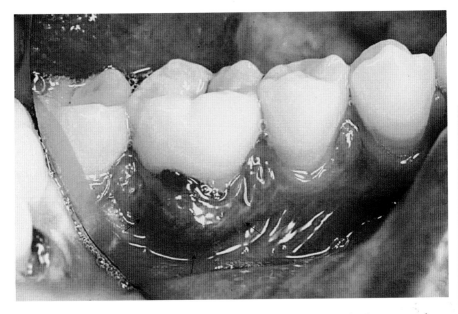

Figure 5.1 Periodontal abscess (© Blackwell Publishing 2003. Reproduced with permission from Reference 1)

can still occur if oral hygiene improves before adequate scaling has taken place to remove the organisms (gingival tissue tightens as hygiene improves and stops pus oozing from the pocket).

Clinical features

Clinical features of a periodontal abscess, which may subside and recur, include:

- Swelling (sometimes localised, sometimes the whole side of face)
- Redness
- Pain
- Pus discharge (in later stages)
- Appears as a *radiolucent* (transparent) area on X-ray

Treatment

Treatment depends on the severity of the periodontal abscess. Short-term treatment includes:

- Hot salt water mouthrinses

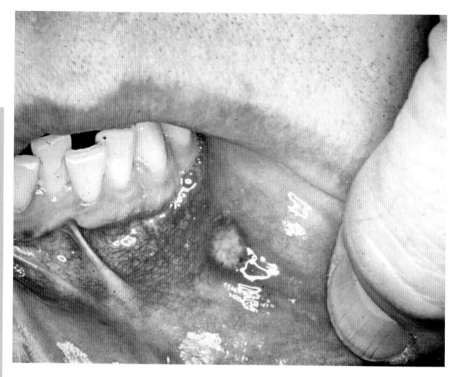

Figure 5.2 Mouth ulcer (*apthous ulceration*) (© Paula Farthing. Reproduced with permission from Reference 2)

- Antibiotics (often required)
- Drainage – through deep scaling, or incision (occasionally required)

Long-term treatment includes:

- Regular deep scaling (ultrasonic scaler) and irrigation (chlorhexidine)
- Extraction (last resort)

MOUTH ULCERS (*APHTHOUS ULCERATION*)

A mouth ulcer (Figure 5.2) is a painful open sore inside the mouth caused by a breach in the *oral epithelium*. Some patients suffer repeatedly for no apparent reason. Mouth ulcers are not contagious.

Aetiology

The causes of mouth ulcers are not fully understood, but predisposing factors include:

- Trauma (from cheek biting, tooth brushing and hard foods)
- Genetic susceptibility
- Reaction to chemicals (e.g. *sodium lauryl sulphate* in toothpaste)
- Vitamin deficiency
- Hormonal (some women develop ulcers prior to menstruating)
- Gastrointestinal disease (e.g. *Crohns*, *ulcerative colitis*, *coeliac*)
- Emotional stress
- Immunodeficiency (e.g. HIV)

Clinical features

Clinical features of mouth ulcers include:

- Painful sores on any part of the mouth's soft tissues. Sores can range in size from a few millimetres (*minor*) to 1 cm or more (*major*). Major sores can leave scarring.
- Can occur singly or in clusters.
- Should heal after 7–14 days – but if no improvement is seen, the dentist should consider referral to a consultant for investigation; an ulcer that does not heal can be a sign of more serious disease, such as diabetes or oral cancer.

Treatment

Treatment of mouth ulcers includes:

- Pain relief (e.g. throat sprays)
- Protection from infection (consider chlorhexidine)
- Avoidance of spicy, acidic or sharp foods
- Good, well-balanced diet
- Control stress
- Toothpaste free of sodium lauryl sulphate

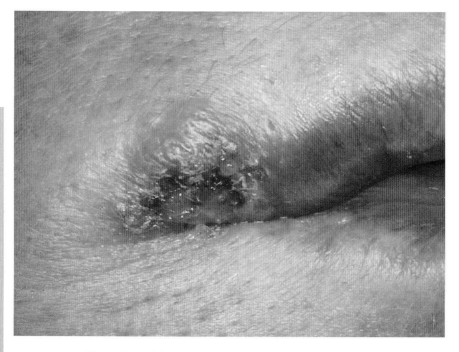

Figure 5.3 Cold sore (*herpes labialis*) (© Professor M.A.O. Lewis, Cardiff University. Reproduced with permission)

COLD SORES (*HERPES LABIALIS*)

Cold sores (Figure 5.3) are very common in the UK and most people are infected in early childhood, often by close contact from a relative (kissing). When a small child is first infected, the disease can present as an acute and unpleasant illness (see acute herpetic gingivostomatitis).

Aetiology

Cold sores are caused by infection with the *herpes simplex* virus (which can live throughout life and reactivate) at nerve endings.

Clinical features

Clinical features (*and contagious stages*) of cold sores include:

1. Tingling in the area of eruption
2. A small, raised blotch that forms blisters

3. Blisters collapse – causing *weeping*

4. Scab – blister dries and heals

5. Contact with others (usually mouth) leads to spread of virus

Treatment

Treatment of cold sores includes:

- Antiviral cream – should be applied at the initial *tingling* stage before clinical signs appear. Scratching or close contact with others (particularly young children) should be avoided.

- Severe cold sores can be treated using systemic antiviral drugs.

What reactivates the virus?

The virus is often reactivated by the following:

- Illness (e.g. colds, flu, AIDS).

- Emotional stress.

- Menstruation.

- Bright sunlight (which explains why people develop cold sores whilst on holiday).

- Extreme cold weather.

- Fatigue and physical injury.

ACUTE HERPETIC GINGIVOSTOMATITIS

Acute herpetic gingivostomatitis (Figure 5.4) is how the *herpes simplex* virus can present in babies and small children, and it is occasionally seen in adults who have lowered immunity.

Aetiology

Acute herpetic gingivostomatitis (like herpes labialis) is caused by infection with the *herpes simplex* virus.

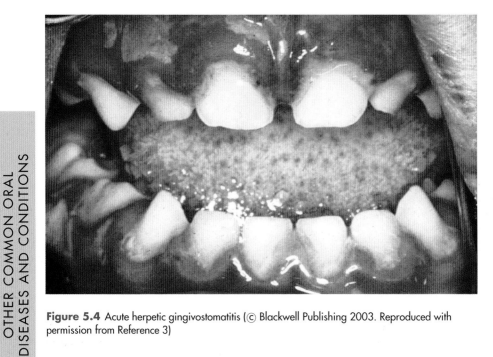

Figure 5.4 Acute herpetic gingivostomatitis (© Blackwell Publishing 2003. Reproduced with permission from Reference 3)

Clinical features

The herpes simplex virus may be mild and produce few symptoms, or may be severe with widespread ulceration. Clinical features of acute herpetic gingivos-tomatitis include:

- Small vesicles (blisters), which rupture and produce ulcers, appear in the mouth and/or throat.
- Sudden onset of feeling unwell and irritability.
- Refusal to eat, causing dehydration.
- Dribbling – as too painful to swallow saliva.
- General malaise: fever, coated tongue, swollen tongue and foul breath.

Treatment

Acute herpetic gingivostomatitis is treated as a flulike illness, by:

- Rest – infants may require hospital treatment to restore fluids if they refuse to drink.

- Frequent drinks, soft foods.

- Mild analgesics.

- Chlorhexidine mouthwash (for adults).

- Gentle oral hygiene.

- Antiviral drugs (may be prescribed in severe cases).

NECROTISING ULCERATIVE GINGIVITIS (NUG)

NUG (Figure 5.5), also known as *Trench mouth* or *Vincent's angina*, is one of the most unpleasant acute illnesses to affect the oral cavity, and can make a patient feel extremely ill.

Aetiology

Causes of NUG are not fully understood – various microorganisms are involved, mainly anaerobic bacteria – the principle bacterium being *treponema denticola*[5], which is capable of invading oral tissues. NUG was common in the trenches during the First World War (hence the term *Trench mouth*) and, although not contagious, tends to occur in communities whose resistance is weak due to ill health or poor environmental conditions.

Today, NUG is most common in young adults between 13 and 25 years old, and often associated with students who have recently moved away from home and have started to look after themselves. Poor diet, smoking, drinking and late nights seem to be common factors. Students are also particularly susceptible during exam time when stress levels are high. Approximately 96% of sufferers smoke – smoking is not a cause but seems to add to risk (M. Midda, personal communications).

NUG is also widespread in patients with systemic conditions that lower resistance (e.g. AIDS). Initial lesions often occur in areas of localised stagnation such as around gingival flaps of erupting wisdom teeth, or recently traumatised gingivae in patients with poor oral health.

Clinical features

Clinical features of NUG include:

- Sudden onset and rapid development.

- Painfully inflamed gingivae, ragged *sloughing ulcers* (easy to diagnose) as bacteria invade the tissues.

OTHER COMMON ORAL
DISEASES AND CONDITIONS

(a)

(b)

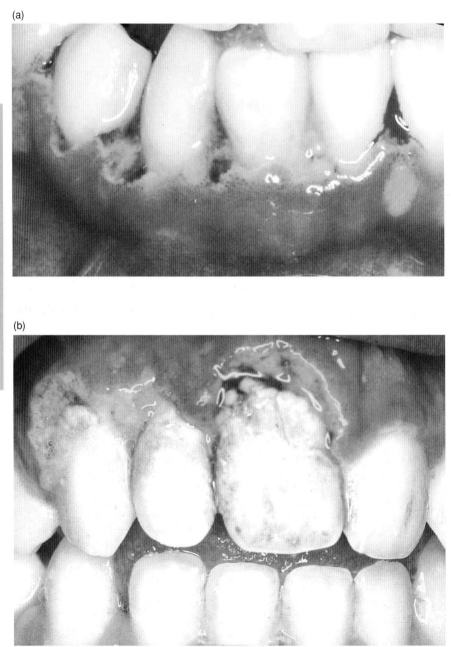

Figure 5.5 (a & b) Necrotising ulcerative gingivitis (NUG) (© Blackwell Publishing 2003.
Reproduced with permission from Reference 4)

- Acute inflammation and bleeding.

- Halitosis. Patients often complain of a metallic taste.

- Swollen glands, temperature and general malaise (occasionally).

- Occurs most frequently during winter months (reason unknown).

- Destruction of tissues when no treatment is available – patients who have repeated attacks often exhibit permanent loss of interdental papillae.

Treatment

Treatment of NUG depends on its severity, but should be rapid to prevent the destruction of the interdental papillae, and includes:

- Antibiotics (*metronidazole*), or penicillin for pregnant patients.

- Thorough scaling using an ultrasonic scaler – this treatment can be delayed until pain permits.

- Hydrogen peroxide mouthwash – for its oxygenating effect (kills anaerobic bacteria). Chlorhexidine should not be used until the initial infection has cleared; thereafter, it may be used to aid oral hygiene procedures.

- Emphasis on excellent oral hygiene procedures – soft, gentle toothbrush for early treatment.

- Cease smoking.

- Plenty of rest to reduce stress levels.

- Regular follow-up scaling and reinforcement of oral hygiene procedures.

- Surgical re-contouring of gingivae when NUG has healed (occasionally required).

- Encourage patient to have a healthy, well-balanced diet (plenty of fresh fruit and vegetables).

OTHER COMMON ORAL
DISEASES AND CONDITIONS

AGGRESSIVE PERIODONTITIS (AP)

AP (Figure 5.6) describes the severe inflammation and rapid bone and connective tissue loss that predominantly occurs in young people aged between 25 and 35 years olds (who otherwise have clean mouths).

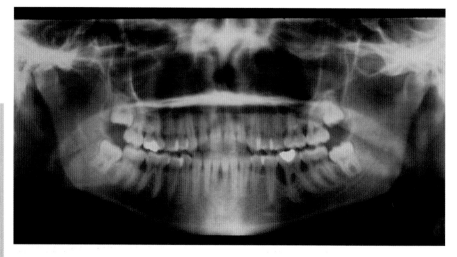

Figure 5.6 Aggressive periodontitis (AP) (© Dr Nicola West, Bristol University. Reproduced with permission)

Aetiology

Causes of AP are not fully understood, but several particular types of bacteria and the *Epstein–Barr virus* (EBV) are commonly found in mouths where AP is present[5]. There may also be some association with poor health, depression or systemic disease such as diabetes. Some patients also seem to have a hypersensitivity to certain bacteria.

Clinical features

Clinical features of AP include:

- Severe and rapidly advancing *lesions* (abnormal tissue). Lesions are frequently generalised, with all teeth affected to a greater or lesser extent.
- Acute inflammation in active phases.
- *Epulis-like* swellings on the gingivae (occasionally).
- Deep pocketing.

Treatment

Treatment of AP includes:

- Regular, thorough scaling (often initially under local anaesthetic)

- Excellent maintenance of oral health by patient
- Systemic antibiotics (occasionally required)

LOCALIZED AGGRESSIVE PERIODONTITIS (LAP)

LAP is a rare form of AP that occurs around the permanent teeth (usually adolescents).

Aetiology

The cause(s) of LAP are unknown, but it is thought to be genetic (siblings are often affected), and associated with specific bacteria causing *neutrophil* (white blood cell) malfunction[5].

Clinical features

Clinical features of LAP include:

- Localisation around first molars and incisors, particularly in teenagers.
- Extent of destruction bears no connection to the oral hygiene of the patient, gingival inflammation is frequently low.
- Racial connections – often seen amongst members of the Afro-Caribbean population.
- *Rapid episodic bone loss* (occurs in bursts of activity).

Treatment

Treatment of LAP includes:

- Systemic antibiotics – either tetracycline, or more commonly a combination of amoxicillin and metronidazole to eradicate associated organisms.
- Surgery (occasionally).

Remember! As with all periodontal diseases, other factors (i.e. immunity, inheritance and host response) are also involved in LAP.

OTHER COMMON ORAL
DISEASES AND CONDITIONS

ORAL CANDIDOSIS

Candidosis is caused by the fungus *Candida albicans*. This fungus is commonly present in the oral cavity and usually causes no problems. However, as with many organisms, it can become active when resistance is low. The most common manifestations of the fungus seen by the dental professional are *oral thrush*, *stomatitis* and *angular cheilitis*. It affects young babies, older people and the terminally ill in particular. Asthma sufferers are also prone to thrush, since the steroids in inhalers alter the oral flora. They should be advised to rinse their mouths out with water after using inhalers.

Oral thrush

Oral thrush (Figure 5.7) is treated using antifungal drugs (e.g. Nystatin^{TM} – systemic, pastilles or oral suspension). Clinical features include:

- Thick, white patches (*like curds*) on the tongue, cheeks, lips and palate.
- Red, raw, sore patches remain when the white coating is removed. This feature helps to distinguish thrush from more serious conditions such as oral carcinoma.

Stomatitis

Stomatitis is a fungal inflammation of the mucous membrane lining of the mouth, and may involve the cheeks, gums, tongue, lips and roof or floor of the mouth. It is associated with denture-wearing, known as *denture stomatitis* (Figure 5.8), and antibiotic therapy. It may occur post-antibiotics (as drugs kill the bacteria which keep candida under control).

Clinical features

Clinical features of stomatitis include:

- Red, shiny, sore patches, often on the palate (especially in denture wearers).

Treatment

Treatment of stomatitis includes:

- Removal and brief sterilisation of dentures at night, if possible, or leave out for periods in the daytime.
- Avoidance of antibiotics (where practical).

OTHER COMMON ORAL
DISEASES AND CONDITIONS

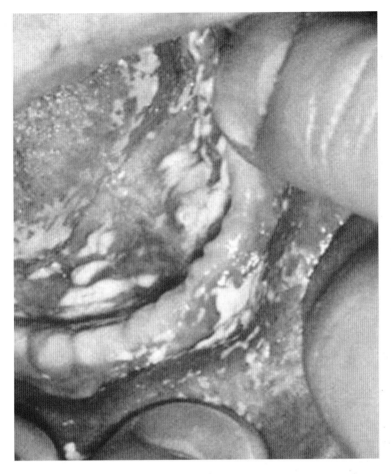

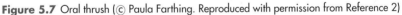

Figure 5.7 Oral thrush (© Paula Farthing. Reproduced with permission from Reference 2)

- Antifungal drugs.
- Gentle brushing of affected areas.

Angular cheilitis

Angular cheilitis (Figure 5.9) causes cracks in the lips, and is usually seen in older people or denture wearers where the mouth *overcloses*. The areas are continually moist, which encourages the proliferation of this fungus.

Clinical features

The clinical features of angular cheilitis are:

- Small, reddened, sore cracks at angles of lips, which either do not heal or continually recur.

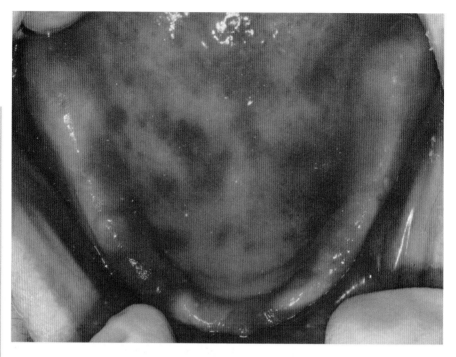

Figure 5.8 Denture stomatitis (© Alison Chapman)

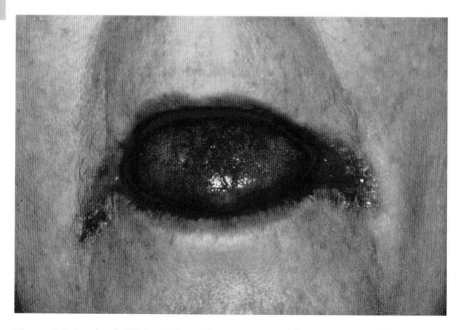

Figure 5.9 Angular cheilitis (© Professor M.A.O. Lewis, Cardiff University. Reproduced with permission)

Treatment

Treatment of angular cheilitis includes:

- Replacement of ill-fitting dentures.

- Antifungal ointment – which must be used for the prescribed length of time (i.e. for several weeks after infection has gone).

WHITE PATCHES (*LEUKOPLAKIA*)

The majority of white patches seen in the mouth are benign, but certain conditions may be pre-malignant or malignant. (It is therefore recommended that all white patches should be sent for biopsy.) There are a number of causes of *leukoplakia* including smoker's keratosis, trauma (such as cheek biting) or aspirin contact next to a tooth.

LICHEN PLANUS

Lichen planus (Figure 5.10) is a systemic skin condition that can also affect the mouth. It principally affects the buccal mucosa, but the tongue, lips and attached gingivae can also be affected. This condition can also be seen elsewhere on the body, appearing as a persistent rash. In rare cases, it can be pre-malignant but not unless changes (such as ulceration and pain) occur. Sometimes there are no oral symptoms, but occasionally they present in the oral cavity and not elsewhere.

Aetiology

The cause(s) of lichen planus are unknown.

Clinical features

Clinical features of lichen planus include:

- Interlacing network of white *striae* (striped skin lesions) commonly seen on the buccal mucosa.

- Red sores – commonly seen on the gingivae (often painless).

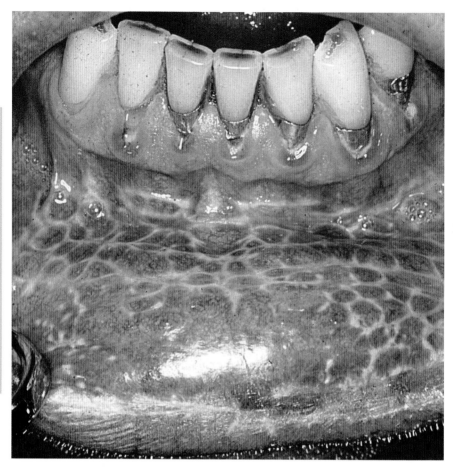

Figure 5.10 Lichen planus (© Blackwell Publishing 2003. Reproduced with permission from Reference 3)

Treatment

Treatment of lichen planus includes:

- Gentle oral hygiene instruction
- Steroid mouthwash (for acute conditions)
- Avoidance of irritants (e.g. spicy or acidic foods)

RED PATCHES

Any unexplained and persistent reddened area in the oral cavity should be referred for investigation as this can also be a sign of oral cancer.

ORAL CANCER (CARCINOMA)

There are around 4000 cases of oral cancer (Figure 5.11) diagnosed in the UK each year[6]. It affects all of the soft tissues in the mouth and salivary glands; and it is a major reason why patients over 50 years old should be screened regularly by a dentist. Early diagnosis improves survival chances.

Aetiology

The causes of oral cancer are debateable, but smoking and alcoholic drinks (especially spirits) are high risk factors as is the chewing of betel nut and similar substances in certain cultures. Research[7] shows that excessive exposure to sunlight increases the incidence of lip cancers, which may present as dark patches or non-healing sores. However, lip cancers are declining through an increased awareness of the dangers of sunlight exposure.

Clinical features

Clinical features of oral cancer include:

- Red patches (more sinister than white patches, especially when *speckled*).
- White patches.
- Lumps or nodules.
- Non-healing ulcers or sores.

Treatment

Treatment of oral cancer includes:

- Surgery.
- Radiotherapy. Side effects of radiotherapy include *xerostomia* (dryness of the mouth), leading to ulceration and increased caries rate.
- Chemotherapy (occasionally).
- Specialised palliative cleaning techniques worked out by oncology care teams, plus the use of mouthwashes and other products. OHEs should be aware of these and consult the patient, relatives and oncology professionals, and can also recommend:
  - Gentle mouth brushing with a very soft brush.
  - Sucking ice chips.

OTHER COMMON ORAL
DISEASES AND CONDITIONS

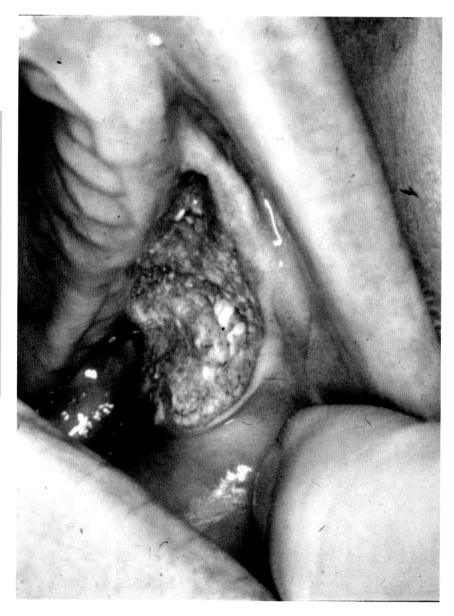

Figure 5.11 Oral cancer (carcinoma) (© Paula Farthing. Reproduced with permission from Reference 2)

Prevention

The following measures should be taken to reduce the risk of oral cancer:

- Cease smoking
- Reduce alcohol intake
- Avoid prolonged exposure to strong sunlight and use sunblock on lips
- Regular dental checks (for early diagnosis)

ACQUIRED IMMUNE DEFICIENCY SYNDROME (AIDS)

Aetiology

AIDS is caused by the *human immunodeficiency virus* (HIV).

Oral manifestations

Oral signs and symptoms of AIDS include:

- Marginal gingivitis, sometimes severe with ulcers.
- NUG – widespread ulceration.
- Oral thrush – recurrent and persistent.
- Herpes simplex virus and *zoster* (*shingles*).
- Swelling of cervical lymph nodes.
- *Kaposi's sarcoma* – rare, late stage. Painless purple swelling usually on the palate.

Treatment

Treatment of these manifestations includes:

- Systemic drugs and palliative care (keeping the mouth as comfortable and healthy as possible).
- Regular, careful scaling.

- Mouthwashes

- Antibiotics.

RECREATIONAL DRUG USERS

Recreational drug users (people who regularly take cannabis, heroin and other drugs not prescribed as part of medical treatment) are particularly prone to oral diseases associated with lowered immunity. OHEs should be aware that patients who repeatedly present with conditions such as NUG, candida and herpetic infections may be using recreational drugs.

SYSTEMIC DISEASES WITH ORAL SYMPTOMS

A systemic disease is one which affects the whole body, such as diabetes, Crohn's disease and colitis.

DIABETES

Diabetes is a common, incurable disease caused by the pancreas failing to produce insulin and characterized by persistent *hyperglycemia* (high blood sugar level). There are two main forms of this disease: *type 1* and *type 2* diabetes.

Type 1 diabetes

Type 1 diabetes, also know as *insulin-dependent diabetes mellitus* (IDDM), often begins in childhood or adolescence and the patient usually requires insulin injections from diagnosis. Patients must stick to dietary recommendations or otherwise face potential complications in later life, including eye problems and difficulties with peripheral circulation leading to soft tissue and organ damage, and periodontal disease.

Type 2 diabetes

Type 2 diabetes, also know as non-*insulin dependent diabetes mellitus* (NIDDM), usually begins in later life and may involve a hereditary factor.

Patients are often unfit and overweight before the disease develops. It can usually be controlled by diet and tablets, but sometimes insulin injections are required. Complications are similar to those associated with type 1.

Oral implications of diabetes

Oral implications (e.g. periodontitis) in both types of diabetes are due to:

- Blood vessel degeneration. Vessels are less able to transport an adequate blood supply, which helps repair and maintain tissue.

- Altered collagen metabolism – the body is less able to produce good quality collagen for adequate tissue repair and maintenance.

- Certain types of white blood cells become less attracted to sites of infection and their function of engulfing and destroying bacteria. Therefore, diabetics are less able to fight infection.

Research shows that bringing periodontal disease under control may also improve the control of diabetes[8].

OTHER COMMON ORAL DISEASES AND CONDITIONS

CROHN'S DISEASE AND COLITIS

These diseases sometimes show oral manifestations, since in some unfortunate patients, the whole of the digestive system, including the mouth is affected. Patients show signs of gingivitis and severe ulceration (despite good oral hygiene in many cases).

SELF-ASSESSMENT

1. Make a series of *flash cards – one* for each condition. Title each card with the name of the disease and list on one side the causes and main features of the disease, and on the other, the group of patients most likely to be affected and the treatment necessary. Highlight words which you particularly want to remember.

   For example:

   Side 1

   Cold Sores

   Cause (aetiology): Herpes simplex virus – probably acquired in childhood and reactivated by Ill-health, exposure to sunlight, stress, fatigue or injury.

   Clinical features: tingling, blister, weeping and scab.

Side 2

Treatment: Antiviral cream in early stages and avoid close contact with others, particularly small children.

2. Write short notes on the advice you would give to a patient who is at risk from oral carcinoma (presenting either symptoms of smoking, heavy drinking habits, or in whom you notice signs of betel nut chewing).

REFERENCES

1. Sanz, M., Herrera, D., van Winkelhoff, A J. (2003) *The Periodontal Abscess.* In Lindhe, J., Karring, T., Lang, N.P. (Eds): *Clinical Periodontology and Implant Dentistry*, 4th edn, pp. 260–268. Blackwell Munksgaard, Oxford.
2. Farthing, P. (2006) *Oral Medicine and Pathology.* In Ireland, R. (Ed): *Clinical Textbook of Dental Hygiene and Therapy*, pp. 51–69. Blackwell Munksgaard, Oxford.
3. Holmstrup, P., van Steenbergh, D. (2003) *Non-plaque Induced Inflammatory Gingival Lesions.* In Lindhe, J., Karring, T., Lang, N.P. (Eds): *Clinical Periodontology and Implant Dentistry* 4th edn, pp. 269–297. Blackwell Munksgaard, Oxford.
4. Claffey, N. (2003) *Plaque Induced Gingival Disease.* In Lindhe, J., Karring, T., Lang, N.P. (Eds): *Clinical Periodontology and Implant Dentistry* 4th edn, pp. 198–208. Blackwell Munksgaard, Oxford.
5. Galgut, P. (2006) *Current Concepts in Periodontology.* Paper given at Gloucester Independent Dental Hygienists *Practical Periodontics Study Day*, Cheltenham, Gloucestershire, 1 December 2006.
6. Levine, R.S., Stillman, C.R. (2004) *The Scientific Basis of Oral Health*, British Dental Journal, BDJ Books, London.
7. The Oral Cancer Foundation. Available at www.oralcancerfoundation.org.
8. Tilling, E. (2007) *Advanced Periodontitis – Where Do We Go from Here?* Lecture given at Gloucester Independent Hygienists' Study Day, Berkley, Gloucestershire, 16 March 2007.

Chapter 6
Caries

LEARNING OUTCOMES

By the end of this chapter you should be able to:

1. Define *dental caries* and state when it first occurred in the Western World.
2. List the least and most common sites where caries occurs.
3. Explain the progression and development of caries.
4. Draw and give a brief explanation of the *Stephan curve*.
5. Conduct simple experiments to demonstrate how an *acid attack* occurs.
6. Describe studies linking caries to the consumption of fermentable carbohydrate.

WHAT IS CARIES?

Caries is the progressive destruction of enamel, dentine and cementum, initiated by microbial activity at a susceptible tooth surface. *Caries* is a Latin word meaning *decay*.

History and distribution

Caries is a social class-related condition and is one of the most common diseases in industrialised countries. In recent years, there has also been a vast increase in caries in developing countries.

Until the seventeenth century, the UK diet consisted of unrefined whole-foods which wore occlusal surfaces flat[1]. However, subsequent changes in flour-milling methods, which made flour more refined, meant that less chewing was required and caries-prone fissures were not worn away. Eating patterns also began a slow but gradual change. For example: in the reign of Elizabeth I, sugar was imported and consumed by the wealthy. The development of dental

CARIES

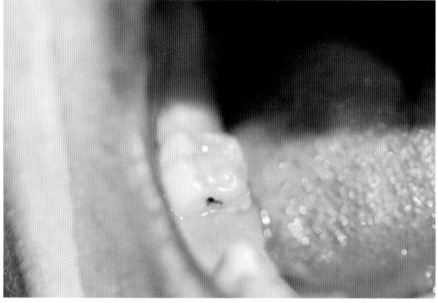

Figure 6.1 Smooth surface caries on lower molar (© Carole Hollins. Reproduced with permission from Reference 7)

caries followed these changes in diet (as sugar became less expensive and widely available to the general population).

In the present-day, sugar consumption has been estimated at around 60 kg per person per year[2] in the UK. However, surveys carried out every 10 years using the DMFT index (decayed, missing and filled teeth)[3] have shown a gradual reduction in caries in children aged between 5 and 12 years. This is largely due to a number of factors, including:

- Improved oral health and dietary education of parents and children.
- Wider availability and use of fluoride toothpaste.
- Regular dental check-ups identifying early problems.

Types of caries

There are three main types of caries:

1. *Smooth surface caries* (Figure 6.1).
2. *Pit and fissure caries* – common in newly erupted teeth (Figure 6.2).

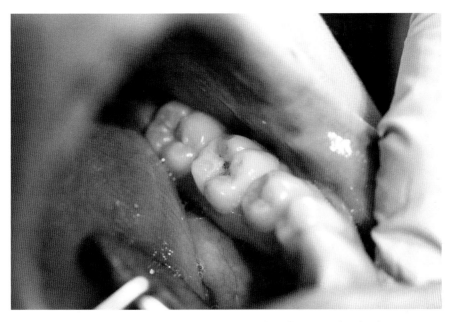

Figure 6.2 Pit and fissure caries in lower molar (© Carole Hollins. Reproduced with permission from Reference 7)

3. *Root caries* – common in the elderly, when root surfaces are exposed (Figure 6.3).

Development of caries

For caries to develop, four factors are required (Figure 6.4):

1. Susceptible tooth

2. Bacterial plaque

3. Bacterial substrate (fermentable carbohydrate, which feeds plaque bacteria)

4. Time

Remember! Susceptible tooth + bacterial plaque + substrate + time = caries.

Aetiology of caries

The normal (resting) pH of the mouth (and plaque) is around 6.8. This is neutral (i.e. neither acid nor alkaline.)

CARIES

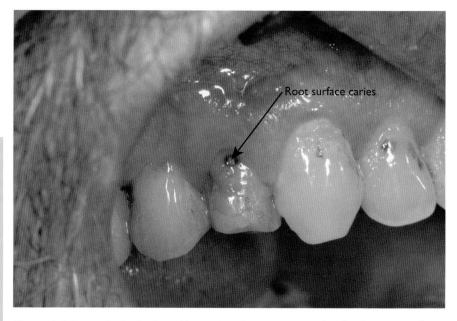

Figure 6.3 Root caries (© Dr Susan Hooper, Bristol University. Reproduced with permission from Reference 7)

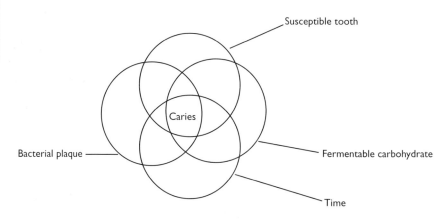

Figure 6.4 Causes of caries (© Ruth McIntosh. Reproduced with permission)

When a susceptible tooth, often newly erupted (where the enamel has not yet matured) is exposed to frequent sucrose intakes, the bacteria present in plaque (most commonly *streptococcus mutans* and *lactobacilli*) produce lactic acid.

The intake of fermentable carbohydrates (starches that break down to sugars in the mouth) causes the pH of the mouth to drop. When it reaches 5.5 (known as *the critical pH*), an acid attack occurs[4].

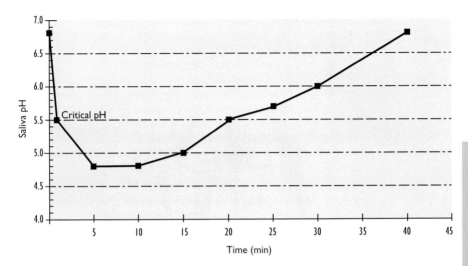

Figure 6.5 The Stephan curve (© Ruth McIntosh. Reproduced with permission)

Acid attack

During an acid attack, *calcium hydroxyapatite* in the enamel begins to dissolve as calcium and phosphate ions leave the tooth and pass into the saliva. This is the first stage in the development of caries, known as *demineralisation*.

Saliva contains bicarbonate ions which have a *buffering effect* (neutralising acid), and if no more sugar is consumed, the calcium and phosphate ions return to the enamel and the pH returns to normal. It takes 30 min to 1 h for this *buffering* to take effect and is known as *remineralisation*. Change in the enamel surface during demineralising and then remineralising is termed the *ionic seesaw* (S. Lockyer, personal communications).

When episodes of demineralisation exceed episodes of remineralisation dental caries occurs.

The Stephan curve (*Remember!*)

The Stephan curve (Figure 6.5) is a graph used to show the development of an acid attack. It illustrates how quickly the pH falls and how long it takes to return to normal.

Stages of caries

The process of caries is described in the stages below:

1. Small pit – an initial break in the enamel extends to the enamel–dentine junction. It can be detected by a probe.

CARIES

CARIES

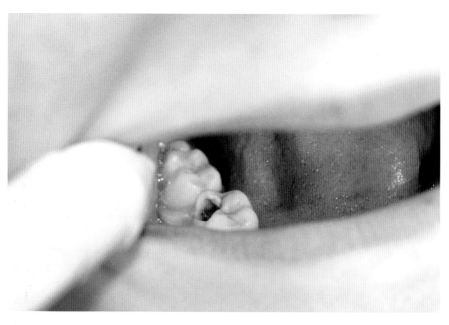

Figure 6.6 Gross caries with collapse of overlying tooth cusp (© Carole Hollins. Reproduced with permission from Reference 7)

2. Blue/white lesion – caries destroys dentine more rapidly than enamel because it is softer. The decay shows through the translucent enamel as a blue/white area.

3. Open cavity – the unsupported enamel collapses (Figure 6.6).

4. *Pulpitis* – when the pulp cavity is reached, pulp becomes inflamed and pain occurs.

5. Apical abscess – infection spreads through the *apical foramen* into the periodontal ligament. Pulp is now dead and the tooth non-vital. Pus forms and swelling develops at the apex of the tooth. (This differs from a periodontal abscess which forms on the side of the tooth).

Common sites where caries occurs

The most common sites where caries occurs are:

- Occlusal surfaces of newly erupted molars and pre-molars
- Contact areas between adjacent teeth
- Exposed root surfaces

Remember! The least common sites for caries to occur are smooth surfaces!

Simple experiments to demonstrate an acid attack

The following experiments are particularly effective for simulating an acid attack to primary school children.

'Coins-in-acid' experiment

Fill a number of plastic cups with fizzy cola, orange juice, orange squash, milk and water. Take five 1 or 2 pence tarnished copper coins and fix them to the cups with clothes pegs, so that half of the coin is immersed in the liquid and the other half remains dry. Leave the coins for an hour and observe the surprising results (as you may have expected cola to be the real 'villain'). The neat orange juice and isotonic drinks will have lowered the pH more than the cola drink. This experiment could also be done for young adults using *alcopops*, high caffeine drinks and isotonic sports drinks.

'Egg-in-fluoride' experiment

Fill an egg cup or one section of an egg box with fluoride toothpaste and plant an egg in it overnight (half the egg should be immersed in the toothpaste). Next day, remove the egg, mark the end which has been free of toothpaste with an indelible pen and wash the toothpaste off. Immerse the egg in an acidic solution, such as white vinegar. Observe what happens.

You should have noticed that bubbles appear on the half of the egg not immersed in the toothpaste, indicating that the shell began dissolving in the acid.

Remember! The role of bacterial plaque in the development of caries is that it:

- Maintains the concentration of acid at the tooth surface
- Resists salivary buffering
- Provides carbohydrate substrate (food for bacteria)

Epidemiology and caries

Epidemiology is the study of the incidence and severity of disease within population groups. A number of studies have contributed to existing knowledge of the cause and development of dental caries.

Two of the most important studies are the Vipeholm and the Hopewood House studies.

The Vipeholm study

One of the most famous of all clinical studies began in 1939 when the Swedish government requested an investigation to determine what measures should be taken to reduce caries in their country. This led to a study of the relationship between diet and caries, which took place at the Vipeholm Hospital near Lund in southern Sweden – an institution for the then-described 'mentally diseased individuals'.

The hospital, with its large number of permanent residents, provided an opportunity for a longitudinal study under well-controlled conditions. A comparable study on human subjects will probably never be repeated, as it would now be regarded as unethical to alter diets experimentally in order to cause caries.

The patients were divided into seven groups: one control and six experimental. Four meals were eaten daily over 1 year, and all patients received a diet relatively low in sugar between meals. During this time, the number of new carious lesions was assessed and found to be very low[5].

After the first year, all but the control group were fed additions of large sucrose supplements in sticky or non-sticky form, either with or in-between meals, and the results noted. The control group, who continued with the basic diet, showed little increase in caries throughout the study. In the experimental groups, the diet was supplemented by sucrose in either drinks, bread, chocolate, caramels, 8 toffees or 24 toffees a day. There was found to be a marked increase in caries in all experimental groups, except when the sucrose drink was taken at mealtimes[5].

The risk of sugar increasing caries activity was greatest if it was taken in sticky form between meals. In the *24 toffees group*, when toffees were eaten between meals, the increase in caries was so great that the supplement was withdrawn[5].

UK dental professionals still base much of their dietary advice upon the results of this study, which ended in 1945, stressing that the frequency of sugar intake should be reduced and confined to mealtimes where possible. They advise against sticky foods and maintain that the rate of development of new disease will fall if their advice is followed.

Conclusions of Vipeholm study (Remember!)
At the end of the study, it was found that[5]:

1. Sugar consumption increased caries activity.

2. The risk of caries was greater if sugar was in sticky form.

3. Risk was greatest if sugar was in sticky form and taken between meals.

4. Increase of caries under uniform conditions showed great individual variation (therefore other factors are involved).

5. Caries incidence reduces on withdrawal of sticky foods from diet.

Hopewood House study

In 1942, an eccentric and wealthy Australian businessman transformed Hopewood House, a country mansion in Bowral, New South Wales, into a home for children of low socioeconomic backgrounds. Since this entrepreneur attributed his own improvement in health to dietary habits, he stipulated that the children should be raised on a natural diet excluding refined carbohydrates.

This environment provided the ideal opportunity for a dental study to take place, and at the time of the study 81 children were living in Hopewood House. They were well fed, well clothed and had daily, supervised exercise. All the children previously had poor oral hygiene, as this aspect of their health was not attended to and there was no fluoride in the drinking water.

Conclusions of Hopewood House study (Remember!)
At the end of the study, it was found that[6]:

1. 63 of the 81 children were caries-free.

2. No child had more than six lesions.

3. All lesions were small.

4. Rates of initiation of new lesions and progress of established lesions were very much below the rates of the general population.

5. The difference between these children and the general population was the absence of refined carbohydrate.

6. Upon leaving Hopewood, their caries rate rose to the same as the general population.

Other evidence-based studies (*Remember!*)

Other studies that show the relationship between sugar consumption and caries include:

- *Toverund* – a Norwegian World War II study when sugar was in short supply. There was a drop in the caries rate.

- *Tristan da Cunha* – a remote, untouched island in the South Atlantic until the 1940s when a fish canning factory was built. Jams, cakes and sweets were

CARIES

imported following an increase in the islanders' wealth. Prior to this event, islanders ate only what they grew or caught themselves. A survey in 1962 noticed that caries incidence had tripled since 1937, due to increased sugar consumption (M. Midda, personal communications).

- *Gnotobiotic* (germ-free) rats – a laboratory study in which rats were fed varying amounts of sugar and their caries rate noted. It was found that germ-free rats fed on high levels of sugar did not develop caries[5] – proving the need for bacteria to be present for caries to develop.

- Sweetened medicines – various studies of children on long-term medication have shown that sugared medicines cause higher caries rates[6].

SELF-ASSESSMENT

1. Define *caries* and state when it first occurred in the Western World.
2. Briefly describe the caries process. Discuss the evidence that relates sugar consumption to dental caries.
3. List the four prerequisites for the development of caries.
4. What role is played by bacterial plaque in the development of caries?
5. List the three main types of caries.
6. Briefly explain the meanings of *demineralisation* and *remineralisation* and an acid attack.
7. List the least and most common sites where caries occurs.
8. Explain the Stephan curve (brief paragraph) and draw it from memory.
9. Briefly describe the Vipeholm and Hopewood House studies and list their conclusions. Name four other studies as evidence that refined sugar causes caries.

REFERENCES

1. Griffiths, J., Boyle, S. (1993) *Colour Guide to Holistic Oral Care, A Practical Approach*, 4th edn. Mosby Year Book Europe, London.
2. Kiple, K.F., Omelas, K.C. (2000) *Cambridge World History of Food*. Cambridge University Press, Cambridge.
3. Office for National Statistics (2004) *2003 Dental Health Survey of Children and Young People*. Stationery Office Books, London.

4. Levine, R.S., Stillman, C.R. (2004) *The Scientific Basis of Oral Health Education.* British Dental Journal, BDJ Books, London.
5. Fejerskov, O., Kidd, E. (2004) *Dental Caries, The Disease and Its Clinical Management.* Blackwell Munksgaard, Oxford.
6. Health Education Authority (1999) *Sugars in the Diet.* Health Education Authority, London.
7. Hollins, C. (2008) *Levison's Textbook for Dental Nurses*, 10th edn. Wiley Blackwell, Oxford.

CARIES

Chapter 7
Tooth surface loss and sensitivity

LEARNING OUTCOMES

By the end of this chapter you should be able to:

1. Distinguish between the four main types of tooth surface loss (TSL).
2. Describe the causes, features and management of TSL.
3. Recognise the effects of betel nut (*paan*) chewing.
4. Explain the causes and describe the treatment of *sensitive dentine*.

WHAT IS *TOOTH SURFACE* LOSS?

Tooth surface loss (TSL) describes the loss of hard tissue when bacterial action (e.g. *in caries*) is not a factor.

There are four main types of tooth surface loss: erosion, attrition, abrasion and abfraction.

Erosion

Erosion (Figure 7.1) is usually seen on occlusal, palatal and lingual surfaces of anterior teeth and sometimes on cervical margins. Dental professionals are seeing much more erosion in recent years and there are a number of reasons for this, mainly associated with modern lifestyle.

Aetiology

Erosion is almost always associated with high acidity, and can be caused by:

• Diet. Often through frequent sipping of carbonated drinks or regular consumption of citrus fruits/drinks. The recommended '5-a-day' fruit and

(a)

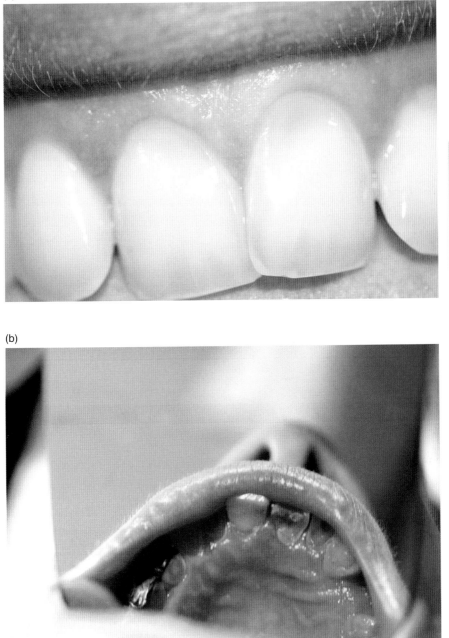

(b)

Figure 7.1 Erosion (a) Erosion on labial surface of upper incisors. (b) Erosion on palatal surface of upper incisors (© Carole Hollins. Reproduced with permission)

vegetable intake in the UK, whilst commendable for general health reasons, can encourage people to eat acid-rich fruits between meals and contribute to erosion if oral hygiene is poor.

- Regurgitation of stomach acids. Commonly seen in anorexics and bulimics, or in people with chronic gastric disorders. Hydrochloric acid is responsible in these cases.

- Acid pollution in the workplace. Now less common in the UK due to improved *Health and Safety* laws, but often occurred in factories (galvanising, pickling, engraving and battery production) – where acid was in the atmosphere.

Features

Features of erosion include:

- Affected surfaces have a smooth, polished appearance
- Anatomical shape is lost or shallow depressions may appear

Patients commonly affected by erosion

Patients commonly affected by erosion include:

- Teenagers who sip carbonated drinks (30% of 13-year-olds showed signs of erosion[1]).
- Sports players with whom *isotonic* sports drinks have become popular.
- Patients with hiatus hernia/similar disorders which cause acid regurgitation.
- Anorexics and bulimics who vomit regularly.
- People who regularly eat citrus fruits (e.g. grapefruit for breakfast, followed by vigorous and damaging brushing), or drink citrus juices.
- Chronic alcoholics where regurgitation may occur.
- Elderly or medically compromised patients whose saliva is greatly reduced.
- Preschool children (24% of 5 year old children showed signs of erosion[1]).

Management

Management of erosion involves:

- Modifying diet (if diet-related).
- Gentle toothbrushing – allow an hour after consuming acidic foods or drinks.

TOOTH SURFACE LOSS AND SENSITIVITY

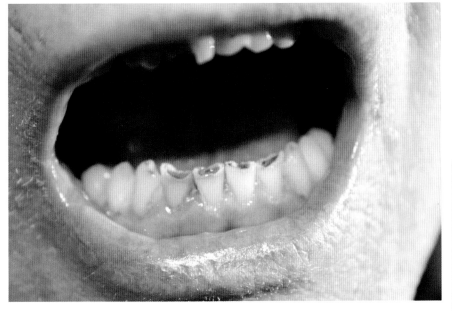

Figure 7.2 Attrition (© Carole Hollins. Reproduced with permission from Reference 2)

- Fluoride application – to increase tooth resistance to acid.
- Reconstruct affected teeth.
- Desensitising agents and toothpastes.

Attrition

Attrition (Figure 7.2) describes the wear seen on the crown of the tooth caused by tooth-to-tooth contact, and is often seen on occlusal or incisal surfaces. It is common in older patients whose teeth have seen more wear and in the deciduous dentition where teeth are relatively soft.

Aetiology

Causes of attrition include:

- *Bruxism* (grinding or clenching).
- Diet (abrasive wholefoods) – seen in Aborigine or Eskimo populations.
- Occupational (rare) – where abrasive dust is mixed with saliva (e.g. mining).

Features

Features of attrition include:

- Matching wear on occluding surfaces
- Shiny facets on amalgam contacts
- Enamel and dentinewear at the same rate
- Possible fracture of cusps or restorations

Patients commonly affected by attrition

Patients commonly affected by attrition include:

- Persistent grinders (often during sleep – a symptom of stress). Some children grind their deciduous teeth away.
- Patients who eat a diet high in abrasive wholefoods (rare in the UK).
- People (e.g. miners) with occupations high in abrasive dust (rare).

Management

The management of attrition is the same as with that of *erosion*, plus the use of a bite-raising splint at night.

Abrasion

Abrasion (Figure 7.3) describes the progressive loss of hard tissue due to mechanical factors other than tooth-to-tooth contact.

Aetiology

Causes of abrasion include:

- Destructive toothbrushing techniques.
- Pipe-smoking.
- Oral and facial piercing, the ring or stud in the piercing can cause wear to the hard and soft tissues of the oral cavity (Figure 7.4).
- Occupational (e.g. pens, hairgrips and tacks frequently held in mouth).
- Saliva combined with abrasive dust (rare, as with *attrition*).

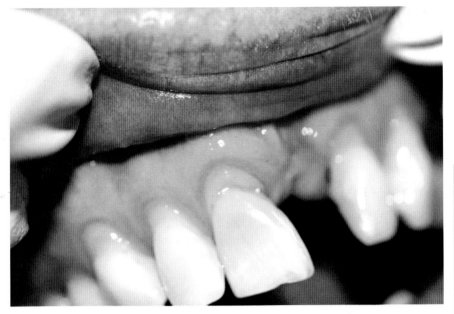

Figure 7.3 Abrasion cavities in upper incisors (© Carole Hollins. Reproduced with permission from Reference 2)

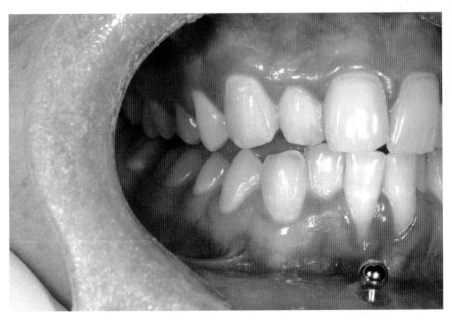

Figure 7.4 Oral/facial piercing causing abrasion to the tooth and gingival recession (© Dr Nick Claydon. Reproduced with permission)

Features

Features of abrasion include:

- Worn, shiny, often yellowy/brown stained areas at cervical margins when aggressive toothbrushing is the cause, or on *biting surfaces* of anterior teeth in pipe-smokers.

Patients commonly affected by abrasion

Patients commonly affected by abrasion include:

- Aggressive tooth brushers.
- People who use very hard toothbrushes.
- People with oral/facial piercing
- Pipe-smokers.
- People who persistently hold foreign objects in the teeth (e.g. hairdressers holding hairpins in their mouths).

Increasingly, younger adults with abrasion are being seen by professionals. This cannot be due to the wear of many years, and it is recognised that the Western diet is less abrasive in modern times. In younger people, it is more likely to be due to *bruxism* (grinding), and over-zealous brushing with large amounts of toothpaste[3]. Some people are obsessed with having 'white teeth' and brush over-enthusiastically several times a day. This can lead to tooth surface loss – the teeth appearing darker – and causing the patient to perpetuate the cycle by brushing even harder.

Management

- Remove piercing or replace with plastic version (as with *erosion.*)

Abfraction

Abfraction (Figure 7.5) describes the pathological loss of tooth enamel and dentine caused by the biomechanical loading of forces (i.e. wear on a tooth caused by irregular bite).

Aetiology

Causes of abfraction include:

- Occlusal forces which flex the tooth substance, inducing chips of enamel that break off.

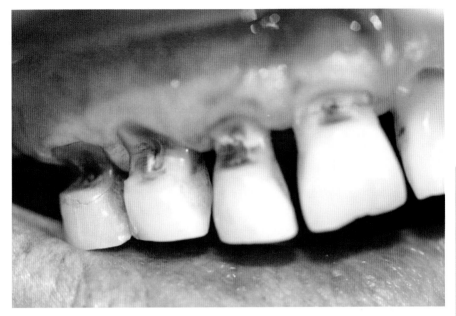

Figure 7.5 Abfraction (© Carole Hollins. Reproduced with permission from Reference 2)

Features

Features of abfraction include:

- Wedge-shaped areas with sharp angled lines at cervical margins or fractured cusps on occlusal surfaces. They can occur alone or in association with toothbrush abrasion. These areas could be misdiagnosed as toothbrush abrasion, but differ as their shape is more acute.

Patients commonly affected

Patients commonly affected by abfraction include:

- Any type of patient, although it is more common in patients with poor tooth alignment. It can be associated with occlusal restorations which may alter the *cuspal movements* and also those with anterior *open bite* and abnormal tongue movement.

Management

Management of abfraction involves:

- Desensitising agents and gentle tooth brushing instruction.

- In severe cases, patients should see a practitioner experienced in this condition for occlusal adjustment. Placing a restoration to reduce sensitivity can help, but if the occlusion is not adjusted this can fail.

SENSITIVITY (DENTINE HYPERSENSITIVITY)

Sensitivity (also known as dentine hypersensitivity) is also an increasingly common dental condition.

Dentine is a highly sensitive tooth tissue, and tooth sensitivity is often complained of by patients who think that they have developed a cavity or lost a filling. On examination, there is often no obvious reason for their pain, although gingival recession is sometimes apparent.

The amount of recession does not appear to be related to the incidence of sensitivity. Patients with large areas of exposed root are often symptom-free, whereas patients with a minimal amount of exposed root sometimes suffer more.

Patients complain of short, sharp, severe episodes of pain sometimes referred to as an 'electric shock'. Common stimuli are cold air and foods (e.g. ice cream), touch by metal (e.g. a fork) and sweet foods (e.g. boiled sweets and toffees)[4]. When *heat* is mentioned as a stimulus, patients complain that the pain develops more slowly but lasts longer.

Sensitivity can result in great distress for patients to the extent that they avoid certain foods and dislike cleaning their teeth with anything but tepid water.

Where does dentine hypersensitivity occur?

The most common sites where dentine hypersensitivity occurs are the buccal and labial surfaces of cervical margins. The teeth most commonly affected are canines and pre-molars (possibly due to over-enthusiastic brushing).

Patients commonly affected by dentine hypersensitivity

Patients commonly affected by dentine hypersensitivity include:

- Young adults (15–35 years old).
- Females. Possibly because they clean their teeth more often and enthusiastically.
- Patients with highly acidic diets (fruit, yoghurt, etc).

- Patients who vomit regularly (bulimics, pregnant women and *hiatus hernia* sufferers).

- Patients with severe occlusal trauma.

- Orthodontic patients (occasionally).

Aetiology

Various theories have been put forward as to the causes of dentine hypersensitivity, but the most likely cause is the stimulation of the tooth pulp, thought to occur when the rate of flow of fluid in *dentinal tubules* changes.

Cold and sweet foods and prodding from metallic objects cause this fluid to contract, but heat results in the expansion of fluid in tubules. Patients who complain of sensitivity to heat describe a pain that develops slowly and lasts longer than pain produced by the other three stimuli. Patients often find that episodes of dentine hypersensitivity occur and then disappear for no apparent reason. The condition often improves over time as secondary dentine is laid down.

Treatment

Dentine hypersensitivity is treated by the application of any of the following products:

- Fluoride varnishes (effectiveness can wear off in time).

- *Siloxane esters* (again, effectiveness can wear off in time).

- Potassium-containing liquids.

- Glass ionomer cements/resins (difficult to apply).

- Composite restorations applied after *air abrasion* of the surface.

- Toothpaste. Seems to be most effective (probably because of its cumulative effect, and abrasive particles such as strontium and potassium blocks tubules).

- Fluoride added to toothpaste. Patients with many sensitive teeth may find relief from using:

  - A fluoride mouthwash (dose: 0.2% solution, 5–10 mL daily – for those over 12 years old).

  - Topical cream (e.g. Recaldent® Tooth Mousse) containing calcium and phosphate which helps to remineralise the tooth surface (not suitable for patients with a milk protein allergy).

SELF-ASSESSMENT

1. What is the term used to describe tooth surface loss caused by mechanical factors? List four causes of this type of tooth wear.

2. Write a short paragraph explaining *attrition* and explaining whom it affects.

3. Write short notes about the effects of acids from food, drink and the stomach (when regurgitated) on the teeth. Include details about people most likely to suffer from these effects.

4. Briefly explain *abfraction*.

5. Which patients complain of sensitive teeth most frequently, what sensations do they usually mention and what seems to trigger their pain?

6. Which teeth are most commonly affected by dentine hypersensitivity, and which areas of the tooth are usually involved?

7. List three ways that you (as an oral heath educator) might advise the patient to reduce sensitivity.

REFERENCES

1. Office of Population, Censuses and Surveys (1993) *1991 UK Census of Population.* HMSO, London.
2. Hollins, C. (2008) *Levison's Textbook for Dental Nurses*, 10th edn. Wiley Blackwell, Oxford.
3. Khan, R. (2006) Eating habits: the effect on the tooth surface. *Smile Journal*, 2(8), 172, Nexus Media Communications, Swanley.
4. Collins, W.J., Walsh, T., Figures, K. (1999) *A Handbook for Dental Hygienists*, 4th edn. Butterworth Heinemann, Oxford.

Chapter 8

Xerostomia

LEARNING OUTCOMES

By the end of this chapter you should be able to:

1. Define *xerostomia*.
2. List the reasons for its occurrence.
3. Explain ways of managing this condition.

WHAT IS XEROSTOMIA?

Xerostomia is excessive dryness of the mouth.

Aetiology

Xerostomia is caused by insufficient oral secretions. A reduction in the amount or flow of saliva, which may occur for various reasons, causes the balance of the mouth to be upset, and contributes to dental disease.

There are a number of reasons why saliva may be reduced or why its flow varies, including:

- Age (saliva production and flow diminish with age).
- Changes in hormone levels (females).
- Prescription drugs. Certain drugs used for: allergies, asthma, depression, diabetes, epilepsy, high blood pressure, inflammatory conditions, infertility, nausea, Parkinson's disease and rheumatoid arthritis.
- Anxiety. Many people will have experienced a *dry mouth* associated with panic – perhaps before a dental appointment or public speaking.

- Acute illness. Diarrhoea and vomiting can cause dehydration, resulting in a reduction in saliva production. Infectious diseases like mumps (inflammation of the *parotid gland*) have the same effect.

- *Mouth breathing*. At night, or in people with malocclusion or chronic sinus problems.

- *Salivary calculi* – calcified stones which are stored in salivary ducts.

- *Sjögren's syndrome*. Associated with autoimmune conditions such as rheumatoid arthritis, in which the lubrication of mucous membranes is drastically reduced. Patients often complain of *dry eyes* as well as a *dry mouth*.

- Radiotherapy (for cancer). Treatment to the head and neck can cause a reduction in flow.

Permanent dry mouth

In some patients, their saliva flow never returns to normal and they suffer greatly from the effects of a permanently dry mouth, which are:

- Increased caries risk. In the elderly, root caries is often the result of xerostomia when gingival recession is present. The root surface does not have enamel protection and is prone to demineralisation.

- Gingivitis (sometimes leading to periodontitis). A reduction in flow diminishes the self-cleansing ability of the mouth when the tongue has no lubrication to help remove stagnating food debris. This leads to more rapid formation of plaque and subsequent inflammation of the gingivae. The oral health educator may have seen the bright red anterior gingivae of people with *lip apart posture*. This occurs because the anterior gingivae are permanently dry.

- Fungal and yeast infections. Organisms (e.g. *Candida*) proliferate in the dry mouth.

- *Glossitis* (sore tongue).

- 'Mouth burning' sensation.

- Ulceration. Particularly affects radiotherapy patients, and can be widespread and exceedingly painful.

- Eating difficulties. Especially painful for radiotherapy patients with ulceration. Imagine trying to eat crisps, chocolate or spicy foods with no saliva and a mouthful of ulcers.

XEROSTOMIA

- Speech difficulties.

- Denture sticking to the mouth.

- Altered oral sensation (mouthwashes and toothpaste may 'burn').

Salivary flow is also greatly reduced during sleep, which is why fermentable carbohydrates should not be consumed late at night after toothbrushing.

Management

Management of xerostomia depends on the cause of the condition. It may not be possible to remove the cause as most people with chronic illness need to continue their drug treatments – so treatment is usually palliative. Patients should mention the problem to their doctor who may be able to change their medication.

Patients should maintain excellent oral hygiene to help with their symptoms. Plaque should be removed thoroughly, teeth cleaned interdentally each day and fluoride toothpaste and mouthwash used. High-fluoride toothpaste is now available in the UK, and is available in two strengths: 2800 ppm and 5000 ppm (by NHS prescription)[1].

Advise Sensodyne Pronamel™, Biotène®, Bioextra® and Kingfisher toothpastes (including aloe vera) and also Biotène® and Bioextra® sprays. Gentle tongue cleansing, with a shaped tongue-cleanser, available from TePe®[2]. Toothpastes that do not contain the foaming agent sodium lauryl sulphate tend to dry the mouth.

Other procedures that may help alleviate symptoms include:

- A diet high in fresh fruit and vegetables stimulates flow. Cut down on sugary snacks.

- Chewing sugar-free gum stimulates flow, but older people may not feel comfortable with this, due to denture wearing or because they were brought up to think that chewing gum was an ill-mannered habit.

- Frequent sips of water or unsweetened drinks (non-alcoholic). Not fruit juice as this is high in acidity.

- Suck small ice chips.

- Biotène® or Bioextra® applied before sleep to moisturise the mouth.

- Lubricate the mouth with non-virgin olive oil or sesame seed oil. Tooth mousse also helps lubrication.

- Preparations containing aloe vera.

Management for radiotherapy patients

Radiotherapy patients (and the chronically sick) need extra special care to alleviate xerostomia. Treatment is usually formulated by medical staff responsible for their care, and may include:

- Frequent, gentle cleaning procedures with specially designed soft swabs and (sometimes diluted) chlorhexidine gluconate mouthwash.
- Use of saliva substitutes available in sprays, toothpastes, gels and mouthwash. Be wary that certain products are artificially manufactured using pig's mucin and may not be acceptable to vegetarians and certain religious groups (S. Bain, personal communications).

These products are effective, but their beneficial effects are usually short-lived.

SELF-ASSESSMENT

1. Define *xerostomia* and briefly describe its effects on the oral cavity.
2. List reasons for its occurrence and patients who might suffer from this condition.
3. Describe treatment to help manage the condition.

REFERENCES

1. Rugg-Gunn, A., Davies, R. (2003) *An Update on Fluoride and Dental Health*. Colgate-Palmolive Ltd., Guildford, Surrey.
2. Tilling, E. (2007) *Xerostomia, Your Patients and You*. Lecture given at Gloucester Independent Hygienists' Study Day, Berkley, Gloucestershire, 16 March 2007.

XEROSTOMIA

ORAL DISEASE PREVENTION

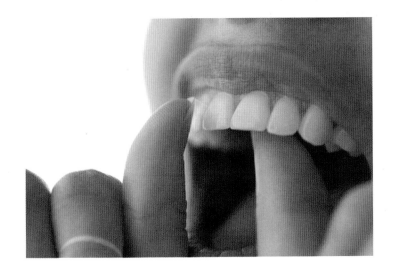

The prevention of oral diseases is now seen as a vital part of dental care in the UK. Increasing numbers of patients are taking responsibility for their own health, by eating a healthy, balanced diet, reducing sugar consumption, giving up smoking and regular brushing and mouth cleansing with fluoridated products.

The dental team also has a vital role to play in the prevention of oral diseases, by providing patients with accurate and up-to-date advice on oral health procedures and products, as well as providing support and encouragement.

This section explores what measures can be taken by both the patient and the dental team in preventing oral diseases.

Chapter 9
Food, glorious food

LEARNING OUTCOMES

By the end of this chapter you should be able to:

1. List the constituents (and their composition, sources and functions) of a balanced diet.
2. Explain the effects of dietary deficiencies on oral health.
3. Define *food additives* and *'E' numbers*.
4. List *food-labelling* laws.

INTRODUCTION

According to the UK Department of Health[1]: 'Eating a healthy, balanced diet which contains plenty of fruit and vegetables and is low in fat, salt and sugar and, based on whole grain products, is important for promoting good health'.

One of the most important roles of the oral health educator (OHE) is to advise patients about diet. Food is the fuel which provides energy for the cells of every living organism to grow, reproduce and eliminate waste; and if the cells of the body are to function efficiently, the following nutritional substances must be available in the correct proportions:

- Proteins
- Carbohydrates
- Fats
- Vitamins
- Mineral salts
- Roughage
- Water

The consumption of the correct proportions of these essential nutrients on a daily basis is known as a *balanced diet*, and is one of the determinants of good oral health.

Proteins

Proteins should comprise approximately 15% of our daily energy intake, and are broken down into amino acids during digestion and absorbed into the body[2]. They are *bodybuilders* and their role is to promote cell growth and repair. Sources of protein include meat, fish, eggs, cheese, milk, vegetables and pulses.

Fats

Fats should comprise approximately 33% of total daily energy intake, and are essential to many body processes, although nutritionists encourage the public to study the quantities and balance of different fats consumed to avoid heart disease and other illness[2]. Fats are found in meat, fish, dairy produce, vegetable oils, nuts and wholegrains. Fats keep the body warm, metabolise cholesterol and act as a reserve source of energy.

Carbohydrates

Carbohydrates should comprise approximately 47% of total energy intake[2]. They are too complex to be absorbed directly by the body and are therefore broken down into smaller units: *monosaccharides*, *disaccharides* and *poly*saccharides[3]. They are found in potatoes, bread, flour, cereals, pasta, rice and sugar. Carbohydrates provide energy.

Remember! The digestion of fermentable carbohydrates begins in the mouth when salivary amylase begins the breakdown of certain carbohydrates to sugars (which can be significant in caries).

Vitamins

Vitamins are a group of complex organic substances that occur in minute amounts in foods. They cannot be synthesised by the body in an adequate supply, and are absorbed unchanged from foodstuffs. The absence of certain vitamins in tissues can cause specific deficiency syndromes[4].

FOOD, GLORIOUS FOOD

Vitamin classification

Vitamins are classified according to whether they are fat-soluble or water-soluble[2].

Fat-soluble vitamins
Fat-soluble vitamins include[2]:

- Vitamin A – found in fish oils, eggs, milk, green vegetables and carrots. It protects against infection, influences changes in epithelial cells and helps eyes see in dim light.

- Vitamin D – found in dairy products, fish and fish oils, and also synthesised from sunlight by the body. It regulates calcium and phosphorus metabolism and helps with the calcification of bones and teeth, protecting against *rickets*.

- Vitamin E – found in nuts, lettuce, egg yolk, wheat germ, cereals, milk and butter. Function is not fully understood, but believed to be concerned with preventing muscle waste, and aiding fertility.

- Vitamin K – found in fish, liver, leafy green vegetables and fruit. It is concerned with blood clotting.

Water-soluble vitamins
Water-soluble vitamins include[2]:

- Vitamins B complex – so called because there are several types (e.g. B6, B12). B vitamins are found in seeds, grains and pulses, and a deficiency can cause anaemia, digestive disorders, skin problems, bleeding gums and glossitis.

- Vitamin C — found in fruit and vegetables. A deficiency can cause scurvy, bone fractures, skin lesions, bleeding gums and damage to the periodontal ligament.

Mineral salts

Mineral salts are also absorbed directly from the diet. They are found in minute amounts in most foods and include calcium, sodium, potassium, phosphorus, magnesium, iron, chloride, iodine and fluoride. They are vital for the healthy function of many organs, provide strength for the skeleton and teeth, and help with nerve and muscle function.

FOOD, GLORIOUS FOOD

Roughage (dietary fibre)

Roughage constitutes substances which cannot be absorbed into the body and pass unchanged through the digestive system, including cellulose from fruit, vegetables, seeds and pulses. Roughage has no nutritional value but is essential for healthy digestion and protection against disorders of the colon and intestines.

Water

Water is, of course, essential for life. It makes up 70% of body weight and is the main dietary constituent. A human being can survive for several weeks without food, but will die in a few days from dehydration.

The average adult needs to consume around 3 litres of water a day (2 litres in drinking and 1 litre from foodstuffs). Even the driest biscuit contains some water.

Food additives *(Remember!)*

A food additive (e.g. *monosodium glutamate*) is a substance not normally consumed as a food by itself, and not normally used as a typical ingredient of food, whether or not it has nutritive value.

Food additives are normally *non-nutrients* (in other words we do not need them to survive), but they are used to improve flavour, colouring, shelf life and convenience in cooking. They generally get a 'bad press', being held responsible for everything from hyperactivity in children to various food allergies. However, it must be remembered that their addition to foods is strictly controlled, and in the EEC, each permitted additive is given an *'E' number*, which signifies that they have been tested and passed for use. This number must be printed on the food label.

Food labelling

There are strict laws governing food labelling, and the OHE should be able to help provide basic advice to patients on how to read labels. Labels in the UK must include[5]:

- Name of food

- Place of origin (if applicable)

- Process used in manufacture

- All ingredients in descending order of weight (at time of manufacture)

FOOD, GLORIOUS FOOD

- Manufacturers' name and address
- Nutritional information (e.g. protein, fat and carbohydrate values)
- Weight (amounts do not have to be listed. Average quantity must be accurate, although weight may vary slightly)
- Date marks (shelf life and 'use by' date)
- Food additives and flavourings ('E' numbers)
- Storage instructions
- Instructions for use

There are exceptions to these rules, where the need for rapid consumption is obvious (e.g. fresh fruit, non-packaged goods).

SELF-ASSESSMENT

1. List the seven constituents of a balanced diet.
2. Write three sentences describing the main sources and function of proteins, carbohydrates and fats.
3. List six vitamins and their sources.
4. Write a brief paragraph explaining the dental implications of vitamin deficiency.
5. List nine mineral salts.
6. Explain what is meant by the terms *food additive* and *'E' number*.
7. List seven laws associated with food labelling.

FOOD, GLORIOUS FOOD

REFERENCES

1. Central Office of Information (2005) *Choosing Better Oral Health, An Oral Health Plan for England*. Department of Health, London.
2. Ross, J.S., Wilson, J.W. (1981) *Foundations of Anatomy and Physiology*, 5th edn. Churchill Livingstone, Edinburgh.
3. Health Education Authority (1999) *Sugars in the Diet: A Briefing Paper*. HMSO, London (out of print).
4. Coultate, T., Davies, J. (1994) *Food, The Definitive Guide*. The Royal Society of Chemistry, Cambridge.
5. Food Standards Agency. Available at www.food.gov.uk.

Chapter 10

Sugars in the diet

LEARNING OUTCOMES

By the end of this chapter you will be able to:

1. Define *COMA* and *NACNE* and list recommendations of the COMA report.

2. Differentiate between *intrinsic, extrinsic* and *milk* sugars, and list the food groups in which they are found.

3. Define hidden sugars and list common sugars found on food labels.

4. Define *artificial sweeteners*, and distinguish between *bulk* and *intensive* sweeteners, stating the sources and uses of each.

INTRODUCTION

Sucrose (table sugar), which is the sugar most commonly used in the UK, provides about one seventh of the average energy (*calorie*) supply in the diet. For about 2000 years, sugar has been extracted from sugar cane in certain tropical countries. In the eighteenth century, it was discovered that sugar could also be extracted from sugar beet.

Approximately one quarter of the sugar consumed in the UK today is in packet or table sugar format, the remainder being derived from its use in manufactured foods and drinks. Sugar consumption has risen steadily in the UK, peaking in 1958 and falling to the present day level, which averages at around 60 kg per person per year (the equivalent of 30 bags of sugar)[1].

Sugar consumption and disease

It is notable that in the wartime years of the 1940s, many foods in the UK were rationed and *luxury foods* were either unobtainable or in short supply. Nutritionists in the two decades following the Second World War were primarily concerned with the effects of food deprivation upon the population, but it was not until the late 1970s that they began to consider that increasing *affluence* can sometimes be more damaging than *deprivation* where health is concerned.

The consumption of sugar in its various forms has long been associated with the development of caries. When fermentable carbohydrates became an important constituent of the Western diet in the seventeenth century, people began to develop dental caries.

Consumption of sugar has also been implicated in a number of systemic diseases (e.g. cardiovascular, cancer and diabetes), as well as contributing to childhood behavioural problems, and detrimental health effects during weaning. However, there is no evidence of a direct link between sugar consumption and the development of these diseases and conditions.

The relationship between sugar consumption and obesity has been given wide publicity in the twenty-first century, perhaps most notably via TV programmes that encourage the audience to study their intake of fats and sugars.

THE COMA PANEL ON DIETARY SUGARS (*REMEMBER!*)

As long ago as 1986, a committee was set up by the UK government to investigate all aspects of diet. The Committee on Medical Aspects of Food and Nutrition Policy (COMA) established the *Panel on Dietary Sugars* to look at the role of sugars in the diet.

In 1989, the panel concluded that the role of sugars in the development of obesity was not clear, but they recommended that when a person is obese, the consumption of non-milk extrinsic sugars (NMES) should be restricted, combined with a reduction in fat intake and regular physical exercise.

The UK Health Education Authority (now the Health Development Agency) set out the panel's findings in a booklet called *Sugars in the Diet*[2].

COMA classification of sugars

COMA distinguishes between sugars held within the cell structure of food (i.e. natural sugars, known as *intrinsic*), and those which have been released from the cell structure (i.e. free or added sugars, known as *extrinsic*). Milk sugars are an exception and also feature in the classification.

Intrinsic sugars

Intrinsic sugars are found in the cell walls of whole fruits and vegetables. They include fructose, glucose and sucrose, which do not begin to break down in the mouth, and are therefore generally less cariogenic than extrinsic sugars.

SUGARS IN THE DIET

Fructose in fruit juices (which may be labelled as having 'no added sugar') is rendered cariogenic by being removed from the plant cell wall. Therefore, fructose in the skin of an apple (which begins absorption in the stomach) is less cariogenic than fructose in apple juice (which salivary amylase begins to break down in the mouth).

Extrinsic sugars (NMES)

Extrinsic sugars are also known as NMES ('enemies' is an easier way to remember these), and include added sucrose, fructose, glucose, dextrose and maltose. NMES are found in confectionery, soft drinks, biscuits, cakes, fruit juices, honey and sugars added to recipes.

Although honey is a natural sugar (comprising glucose and fructose), its consistency facilitates its initial breakdown in the mouth, and it is therefore considered to be cariogenic. Honey is often marketed as a natural 'healthy' food, which it is, but it should be remembered that it has the potential to cause caries when eaten frequently between meals. The same applies to dried fruits (e.g. sultanas and raisins), which parents often give to small children as a snack, thinking that the fruit content renders them safe for teeth, when in fact the drying process in which they undergo during manufacture converts intrinsic sugars into NMES.

Other NMES, often seen on food labels, include syrup, raw sugar, brown sugar, muscovado and cane sugar.

Milk sugars

Milk sugars include lactose and galactose and occur naturally in milk and milk products, such as yoghurt and cheese. They are regarded as less cariogenic than intrinsic sugars because they are accompanied by other essential nutrients (e.g. calcium), which seem to counteract potential damage to teeth.

COMA panel recommendations (*Remember!*)

COMA's recommendations[3] are still regarded as an important guideline for those giving oral health advice in the UK today, and include:

- The consumption of NMES by the population should be decreased and replaced by fresh fruit, vegetables and starchy foods. For adults and children, the average intake of NMES should be limited to 10% of total dietary intake.

- The frequency of sugary snacks and drink consumption should be minimised. Foods and drinks that predispose caries should be limited to main mealtimes. This is especially important for older *dentate* people, children and adolescents.

SUGARS IN THE DIET

- Those providing food for families and communities should seek to reduce the frequency of sugary foods and drinks, and restrict them to mealtimes.

- Schools should promote healthy eating patterns both by nutritional education and by providing and encouraging nutritionally sound food choices.

- Sugars should not be added to bottle foods of infants and small children – sugary drinks should not be given in *feeders* which are in contact with teeth for prolonged periods; and dummies or comforters should not be dipped in sugar or sugary drinks. Weaning foods should be free of (or low in) sugar, including sugars derived from fruit juices and fruit concentrates.

- Bottlefeeding after the age of 1 year should be discouraged, especially for those toddlers who regularly consume soya or infant formula, which contain extrinsic sugars.

- Older people (who have natural teeth) should restrict the consumption of NMES because their teeth are more prone to decay due to root exposure and diminished saliva.

- When medicines are needed (particularly in the long-term), *sugar-free* formulations should be prescribed and selected by parents and doctors, respectively. In addition, food manufacturers should produce *low sugar* or *sugar-free* alternatives to existing sugar-rich products, particularly those for children.

THE NACNE REPORT (*REMEMBER!*)

Oral health educators (OHEs) also need basic knowledge of the National Advisory Committee on Nutritional Education (NACNE) report[4] which was published in 1983, yet is still relevant today.

This report outlined links between diet and a range of conditions and diseases, including caries and coronary heart disease. It suggested, for the first time and 6 years ahead of COMA, quantitative dietary targets for the prevention of diseases associated with affluence.

The targets were short-term (to be achieved by the end of the 1980s) and long-term (to be achieved by the end of the twentieth century). It sets guidelines for the population to reduce fats, salt and sugars, and to increase consumption of oily fish, fibre and fruit.

Frequency of sugar consumption

The dental profession has been aware for over half a century that the *frequency* of sugar intake is far more significant in the development of caries than the *amount* consumed at any given time.

SUGARS IN THE DIET

Patients will often ask and be surprised about the amounts of sugar in different foods and drinks. It is therefore helpful to be able to give an information sheet, setting out these amounts. When producing an exhibition or display, points about reducing sugar consumption can be emphasised by setting out a table of common snacks and putting sugar lumps or small bowls of sugar beside each to show the amount in each snack or drink.

OHE advice to patients on sugar consumption

OHEs should be able to advise patients on the following topics, in order to reduce their intake of sugars.

Reduce all snacks

Particularly those containing sugar. It is important to give the same advice as other health professionals (such as dieticians and health visitors), who are concerned with other aspects of health, such as obesity.

Find healthy alternatives

In the past, the dental profession has suggested that plain crisps, peanuts and cheese are tooth-friendly alternatives to sweets, biscuits and confectionery. When reading labels, it can be seen that some nut snacks contain hidden sugars, and this should be pointed out to patients.

OHEs must also be aware that patients may be told by other health professionals to avoid these foods for other health reasons. Advice must also be balanced by awareness that people (particularly schoolchildren and adolescents) require frequent intakes of carbohydrates to sustain energy. In such cases, it is a good idea to suggest frequent snacks such as pasta, bread and toast, breadsticks, fruit and raw vegetables.

Identify 'hidden' sugars

Many people still associate sugar with white refined sucrose (table sugar), although public awareness of hidden sugars is growing with the current trend towards healthy eating. It is important to be able to identify hidden sugars (e.g. *glucose, fructose, dextrose, maltose, lactose* and *molasses*), and advise patients to look for them on food labels.

Avoid adding sugar

It is still common practice to add sugar to tea, coffee and cereals. This is a hard habit to break, particularly when started in childhood. OHEs should advise pregnant women and parents of young children that adding sugar to food can contribute to obesity and heart disease as well as caries and behavioural disorders.

Consider using sugar substitutes

The use of artificial sweeteners is increasing as the public becomes more diet-conscious, since their low calorific value means that they are virtually non-cariogenic and non-fattening. Sweeteners can be of synthetic or natural origin (e.g. *xylitol*, a plant extract).

Sugar substitutes

EEC permitted sweeteners in the UK fall into two groups: *bulk sweeteners* and *intense sweeteners* (identified by 'E' numbers on food labels). Many people are concerned about the safety of sugar substitutes, as the public becomes more informed about food additives.

In 1995, the EEC directed:

- The justification of sweeteners in energy-reduced, non-cariogenic foodstuffs and food without sugars.

- The extension of the numbers of sweeteners used in the UK, ruling that maximum intake levels should be stated on labels.

- Sweeteners may not be used in foods intended for infants and young children.

- Warning labels must be used.

- Sugars must be indicated in the list of ingredients.

Bulk sweeteners

Bulk sweeteners replace sugar weight-for-weight, look like sugar and are used in foods where bulk is needed (e.g. in cooking, particularly for diabetics and also in medicines). They can supply similar energy levels as sucrose, and are equally (or slightly less) sweet. They are not readily used by oral bacteria, and acid attacks do not occur unless they are used in conjunction with extrinsic sugars.

The main bulk sweeteners used in the UK are:

- *Sorbitol* (E420)

- *Mannitol* (E421)

- *Isomalt* (E953)

- *Malitol* (E965)

- *Lactitol* (E966)

- Hydrogenated glucose syrup

SUGARS IN THE DIET

- *Xylitol* (E967) – particularly important since it is non-cariogenic. Future research should establish whether it can help to prevent caries in children, when given to pregnant mothers in toothpaste and chewing gum[3].

Remember! The names of these bulk sweeteners, but not the 'E' numbers.

Intense sweeteners

Intense sweeteners have no nutritional value, no bulk and no calories. They are usually manufactured in the form of minute pellets, are up to 300 times sweeter than sucrose and, like bulk sweeteners, are not a substrate for oral bacteria.

The main intense sweeteners used in the UK are most readily recognised by the public as they are used to sweeten tea and coffee and are popular with dieters:

- *Acesulfame K* (E950)
- *Aspartame* (E951)
- *Saccharin* (E954)
- *Thaumatin* (E957)

SELF-ASSESSMENT

1. Define COMA, list the recommendations of the COMA panel and the year they were made.
2. Define NACNE, the year the report appeared and the issues it addressed.
3. What is the role of the OHE in advising patients about sugar consumption?
4. What is an intrinsic sugar and where is it found?
5. What is an extrinsic sugar and where is it found?
6. Name two milk sugars and state where they occur.
7. How might you advise a patient to recognise hidden sugars on food labels?
8. What is a sugar substitute? Name the two different types.
9. List six bulk sweeteners and state when they are used.
10. List five intense sweeteners and state when they are used.
11. What is the special property of xylitol?

REFERENCES

1. Kiple, K.F., Omelas, K.C. (2000) *Cambridge World History of Food*. Cambridge University Press, Cambridge.
2. Health Education Authority (1999) *Sugars in the Diet*. Health Education Authority, London.
3. Fejerskov, O., Kidd, E. (2004) *Dental Caries, The Disease and Its Clinical Management*. Blackwell Munksgaard, Oxford.
4. National Advisory Committee on Health Education (1983) *A Discussion Paper on Proposals for Nutritional Guidelines for Health Education in Britain*. Health Education Council, London.

SUGARS IN THE DIET

Chapter 11
Fluoride

LEARNING OUTCOMES

By the end of this chapter you should be able to:

1. Define *fluoride* and state where it occurs naturally.
2. Quote names, dates and places of historical fluoride events.
3. List the benefits of fluoridated water and ways that fluoride strengthens teeth.
4. Differentiate between *systemic* and *topical* administration of fluoride.
5. Define and describe *fluorosis*, why it occurs and the treatment for fluoride overdose.
6. List the commercial products containing fluoride.
7. State the recommended dosage of fluoride in toothpaste for children and adults. Quote recommended instances and doses for fluoride tablets and drops for children.
8. List the arguments *for* and *against* water fluoridation.
9. Explain the significance of the Knox and York reports.

WHAT IS FLUORIDE?

Fluoride is a compound of the naturally occurring element fluorine, and is a part of a group of chemicals known as halogens.

Where is it found?

Fluoride is found:

- Naturally (e.g. in water, soil, rock, air and many plants)
- In our diet (e.g. fish bones, tea and beer)

Fluoride is an essential component of body fluids and soft tissues. Most fluoride in the body is deposited in the bones and teeth.

Fluoride is added to most toothpaste, and has been proven to reduce the incidence of tooth decay dramatically over the last 30 years in the UK[1]. The addition of fluoride to toothpaste has been the biggest single development in the prevention of dental caries, causing a reduction in incidence by 20–30%[2].

Research has also shown[3] that the reduction in caries is found when toothpaste is regularly used at 1500 parts per million (ppm is the accepted method of measuring fluoride in water: 1 ppm = 1 mg/litre).

Fluoride is also used in:

- Rat poison, insecticide and in certain industries (fertilizer and aerosols).

- Certain drugs (e.g. steroids and tranquillisers).

Facts about fluoride

Here are some useful facts about fluoride:

- *Calcium fluoride* is the form that often occurs naturally in water supplies.

- *Sodium fluoride* is the form used to artificially raise levels in drinking water.

- Optimum level in drinking water = 1 ppm.

- The fluoridation of water is the adjustment of the amount of fluoride in water supplies to 1 ppm.

- Fluoride is readily absorbed from the stomach and rapidly excreted via the kidneys, mostly in urine, and also through sweat and faeces. Traces can be found in hair, tears, breast milk and saliva.

- 50% of fluoride in the body[3] is stored in the bones and teeth. It can help to alleviate conditions such as osteoporosis and helps developing teeth become more resistant to caries.

FLUORIDE

History of fluoride

It is useful for OHEs to know a little about the history of fluoride.

1892 (UK)

Sir James Crichton Browne was the first dentist recorded to remark upon the possible connection between fluoride and the incidence of caries[2].

1901 (Colorado Springs, USA)

Dr F. McKay observed 'mottled enamel' in patients, characterised by minute white, yellow or brown spots scattered over tooth surfaces. In certain American states, a relationship between tooth staining and the presence of naturally occurring fluoride in water was observed[3].

1930s (USA)

McKay and Black associated the mottled effect of enamel and low incidence of caries with high levels of fluoride in drinking water[3]. The term *dental fluorosis* was applied to the condition of intrinsic staining caused by fluoride ingestion at over 2 ppm during tooth formation.

1930–1940 (South Dakota, USA)

Dr H. Trendley-Dean carried out research in South Dakota, Wisconsin and Colorado. He showed that the severity of tooth mottling was affected by the concentration of fluoride in the water, and that a near maximum reduction in caries occurred when water contained 1 ppm[2]. He therefore deduced that 1 ppm was the optimum level. His research is still in use today.

Remember! The names and dates of McKay and Trendley-Dean.

1945 (Michigan, USA)

Sodium fluoride was added to drinking water in Grand Rapids, Michigan, and resulted in a 50% reduction in caries incidence[2].

1955 (UK)

Kilmarnock, Watford and part of Anglesey had 1 ppm fluoride added to the drinking water. After 5 years, a 50% reduction in caries was found[2]. However, local opposition in Kilmarnock halted fluoridated water, and the caries rate rose steadily to previous levels.

1964 (UK)

In 1964, water in Birmingham and Newcastle became fluoridated. (Birmingham discontinued its fluoridation in 1998.) Strathclyde decided to fluoridate its water supply but this was opposed (partly on the grounds that it could cause cancer), and in a famous case the High Court of Scotland ruled that although water fluoridation was safe and effective, due to a legal technicality, Lord Jauncy found in favour of the opponent[4].

Remember! The term Jauncy used in the trial was 'ultra vires', meaning 'outside of his power'.

1985 (UK)

The *Strathclyde case* led to the establishment of a committee, led by Professor Knox to investigate the possible harmful effects of fluoride. The *Knox report*, published in 1985, found no evidence that fluoride when added to water causes cancer[5].

2000 (UK)

A systematic review (carried out by the University of York) was commissioned by the chief medical officer of the Department of Health, who requested: 'an up-to-date expert scientific review of fluoride and health'. The main conclusions of this review were:

- Fluoride reduces the prevalence of caries.
- A beneficial effect was still evident in nine studies conducted after 1974 (when fluoride was first added to toothpaste).
- Evidence from 15 studies showed that water fluoridation reduces inequalities in dental health across social classes in 5–12-year-olds, using the dmft/DMFT index.
- The prevalence of dental fluorosis increases with the concentration of fluoride in the water.
- No association was found between fluoridated water and bone fractures or bone development problems (29 studies).
- No association was found between water fluoridation and bone, thyroid and all other cancers (26 studies).

The authors of the review were surprised that, given the level of interest surrounding the issue of public water fluoridation, little high-quality research has been undertaken. Any future research into the safety and efficacy of water fluoridation should be carried out with appropriate research methods to improve the quality of the existing evidence base[6].

Benefits of water fluoridation

The safety of water fluoridation is upheld by the Royal College of Physicians, the Strathclyde case and the World Health Organisation (WHO). Benefits of water fluoridation include:

FLUORIDE

- At a concentration of 1 ppm, fluoridation negates the risk of enamel fluorosis and can reduce caries by 50% (with no patient effort and negligible cost)[2].

- Reduction in caries rate lasts throughout life, since the hydroxyapatite of tooth enamel has been replaced by *fluorapatite* in the developing tooth (fluorapatite is more resistant to acid attacks).

- Economic – it is less expensive to fluoridate water than to fill teeth.

- Improves dental health of all who live in a *fluoridated area*.

For example: in the UK, the beneficial effects of naturally occurring fluoride have been shown by comparing North and South Shields. North Shields has less than 0.25 ppm fluoride in its water, while South Shields has up to 2 ppm fluoride. The DMF index shows that South Shields has almost half the caries rate of North Shields[2].

How fluoride works

Fluoride reduces the incidence of caries in the following ways:

- In the developing tooth, calcium hydroxyapatite in enamel is replaced by calcium fluorapatite which withstands a lower pH of 4.5 rather than the normal 5.5. Teeth erupt with shallower pits and fissures when systemic fluoride is given and are more resistant to acid attack.

- Topical fluoride plays a part in ionic exchange, acting as a catalyst and helping to return more acid-resistant crystals to the tooth.

- Fluoride blocks the enzyme systems of plaque bacteria, inhibiting their ability to turn sugars into acids.

- Fluoride has also been shown to remineralise early carious lesions when used topically.

Fluoride administration

Fluoride can be administered in two ways: *systemically* and *topically*.

Systemic administration

Fluoride is administered systemically through drinking water, aiding the developing teeth in children. The fluoride in milk (if added), salt, tablets or drops and *swallowed* toothpaste can also be considered as systemic and works in the same way, being carried to teeth and bones via the blood.

FLUORIDE

Experts argue whether there is any benefit to the unborn child's developing teeth from the mother taking fluoride supplements or drinking fluoridated water during pregnancy. It is thought that about one third of ingested fluoride crosses the placenta, and therefore supplements for pregnant women are rarely recommended.

Topical administration

Fluoride is applied topically to the surfaces of erupted teeth by various means (e.g. toothpastes, rinses, varnishes and gels). Where systemic fluoride is being administered, there can be additional topical effects from sucking tablets.

Fluorosis

Fluorosis occurs when too much systemic fluoride is ingested, and presents dentally as opaque or white areas and lines or flecks on the enamel surface. It is most noticeable in the anterior regions.

In geographical areas where water has high naturally occurring fluoride (in excess of 7 ppm), as seen in parts of India for example, it can result in very unsightly, yellow/brown pitted teeth. In the UK, these opaque or white areas on teeth are not always the result of ingesting too much fluoride but can be due to a number of causes (e.g. enamel faults caused by high temperatures and fever during tooth development).

If a child ingests fluoride in excess, usually by swallowing toothpaste in larger quantities than the recommended 'pea-sized' quantity from a brush, fluorosis can occur. This risk increases in areas where the water is fluoridated or when a child is receiving fluoride supplements. The greatest risk of fluorosis to the permanent incisors is between 15 and 30 months of age, when these teeth are developing.

Children under 3 years should be allowed only a smear of toothpaste on the brush. This is also an age when toddlers, if allowed unrestricted access to toothpaste, may be tempted to swallow paste, and care should be taken to keep toothpastes out of their reach and supervise toothbrushing. Some toothpastes are produced especially for small children and contain lower levels of fluoride. These pastes tend to be given flavours such as strawberry, which makes the risk of swallowing greater. Children under the age of three should be given a smear of toothpaste containing 1000 ppm. Anyone over the age of three should have toothpaste containing 1400–1500 ppm and use a small pea size amount.

Fluoride swallowed in excessive quantities can be extremely toxic, particularly to small children, and if an overdose is suspected, the immediate antidote is for the child to drink milk and be taken to hospital as quickly as possible. Table 11.1 shows the association between levels of fluoride in water and fluorosis (M. Midda, personal communications).

Table 11.1 The association between levels of fluoride in water and fluorosis

Level of fluorosis	PPM in water	Effect on tooth
None	<1 ppm	None
Not significant	1 ppm	No significant mottling and around 50% caries reduction
Very mild	2 ppm	Small white opaque patches
Mild	2–3 ppm	White opaque area involving half the crown
Moderate	3–4 ppm	White opacity of crown and some brown mottling
Severe	>4 ppm	White opacity of whole crown, brown mottling and pitting and hypoplasia

Fluoride availability

As mentioned, fluoride can be obtained from a variety of sources, including water, fluoride varnish, gels, mouthwashes, toothpaste and fluoridated milk, salt, tablets and drops, which are now looked at in more detail.

Water

Ten per cent of the population of England currently receives a water supply which is either naturally or artificially adjusted to the optimum level of 1 ppm[7]. The British Dental Association (BDA), together with the British Medical Association (BMA), and the British Fluoridation Society responded to a Primary Care Trust survey of patients in 2005 by asking the House of Lords to amend a bill on fluoridation of water supplies which was going through parliament. This was passed in July 2005, allowing the fluoridation of water supplies by local authorities in response to public demand[8].

Fluoride varnish (*Remember!*)

The most commonly used varnish is *Duraphat*®, which contains 2.26% of available fluoride (50 mg/mL). It is applied in the surgery and is used for hypersensitivity and caries prevention.

Fluoride gels

Gels (e.g. Gel-Kam® and Omnigel) contain 0.4% *stannous fluoride*, and should be applied daily at home in small amounts after brushing, using a toothbrush, cotton bud or finger. They are used to treat dentine hypersensitivity and early carious lesions (preventing root caries in older people).

Acidulated phosphate fluoride (APF) gels

APF gels are for topical use in the surgery, although they are rarely used in the UK. The gel is applied in a tray system for an optimum period of 4 min ideally at six-monthly intervals. The risk of toxicity is high and so a good application technique is vital to avoid ingestion.

Mouthwashes (*Remember!*)

Mouthwashes can be used daily (0.05% sodium fluoride solution), or weekly (0.2% solution). Daily use is most effective for dentine hypersensitivity and *high caries risk patients*. These mouthwashes are often recommended for patients undertaking *fixed appliance therapy*.

Toothpastes

Ninety-five per cent of toothpastes in the UK contain a fluoride compound (either sodium monofluorophosphate, sodium fluoride or both)[2]. Toothpastes should contain not more than 1500 ppm of fluoride, and patients should be encouraged to spit after brushing and not rinse toothpaste away.

Toothpastes with a greater concentration of fluoride (2800 ppm, on NHS prescription and 5000 ppm, on private prescription) are now available. They are used for adults and adolescents with high caries rates, root caries and fixed appliance therapy on the advice of the prescribing dentist.

Fluoridated milk

Fluoridated milk in UK schools was once advocated as an alternative means of giving fluoride by the *Borrow Milk Foundation* (a registered UK charity). The problem with this mode of administration was the variable uptake for the individual child, since not all children drank milk (which is also only drunk during term-time).

Fluoridated salt

This method is used in Switzerland, Hungary, France and Germany. The promotion of salt has wider health implications and may result in conflict with other health messages.

Tablets or drops

Between the 1970s and 1990s, fluoride tablets and drops were widely recommended by the UK dental profession as an acceptable means of providing systemic fluoride for children with the additional topical benefits. However, the

FLUORIDE

administration of these supplements is no longer considered to be an effective public health measure.

Since the introduction and widespread use of fluoride toothpaste, many experts believe that these supplements (containing sodium fluoride in 0.5 mg and 1 mg concentrations) should only be recommended when there is a medical history indicating that dental treatment is to be avoided wherever possible (e.g. cardiac, haemophiliac, severely physically/mentally disabled patients or patients with a family history of caries).

Points to consider when recommending supplements

If supplements are recommended, the following points should be taken into account:

- Safe amounts of fluoride supplements can only be recommended if the level of fluoride in the water supply is known.

- Maximum benefit likely only if administered between 6 months and 13 years.

- Critical level for fluorosis is between the ages of 15–30 months (the development period of permanent incisors).

- Must not be administered at the same time as fluoride toothpaste.

- If one dose is missed, it must not be doubled the next day.

- Do not use if going on holiday – there may be fluoride in destination's water.

Table 11.2 shows the recommended doses for daily fluoride which maximises the benefits of fluoride, and minimises the risks (M. Midda, personal communications).

Table 11.2 Recommended daily doses for fluoride supplements

Age	Fluoride level below 0.3 ppm	Fluoride level between 0.3 and 0.7 ppm	Fluoride level over 7 ppm
6 months to 3 years	0.25 mg	None	None
3–6 years	0.5 mg	0.25 mg	None
Over 6 years	1 mg	0.5 mg	None

Patients recommended for fluoride supplements

Patients who are recommended to receive fluoride supplements include:

- Children at risk in areas with sub-optimal water fluoride levels.
- Medically/physically compromised children (e.g. children that are not likely to be cooperative to dental treatment and haemophiliacs).
- Children with siblings who have high caries rate.

Arguments for and against the fluoridation of water supplies

Table 11.3 highlights the main arguments for and against the fluoridation of water supplies.

Table 11.3 The main arguments for and against the fluoridation of water supplies

For	Against
1. We should have freedom of choice	1. It is unethical, as it is mass medication
2. Relatively inexpensive	2. Mainly only benefits children
3. It is the safest way of administering fluoride	3. Fluoride is also used as a poison
4. It is the most effective way of reducing caries incidence[5]	4. There are other methods of reducing caries incidence
5. It works systemically and topically	5. Can be found in fish, tea and other foodstuffs for those who want systemic effect and can be administered in toothpaste topically
6. It reduces the necessity for extractions under general anaesthetic; therefore, mortality risks are reduced	6. Its toxicity can lead to stomach upsets, mental and physical disability and cot deaths
7. It is particularly beneficial in reducing caries in children of low socioeconomic groups	7. Can cause fluorosis – it is impossible to regulate how much fluoride children consume
8. The Knox report[5] and York report[6] said that fluoridated water does not cause cancer	8. Some experts have argued that it can cause cancer of the thyroid and bones, for example

FLUORIDE

SELF-ASSESSMENT

1. Write a sentence, explaining what fluoride is, where it is found naturally and where it is used artificially.

2. Briefly distinguish between systemic and topical administration of fluoride.

3. How does fluoride reduce the incidence of caries?

4. What is meant by the optimum level of fluoride?

5. Who carried out extensive research in USA in the 1930s, which forms the basis of our knowledge on mottling today? What is this mottling called and what does the tooth look like?

6. Which year and where was sodium fluoride first added to drinking water?

7. Name three areas in the UK which have in the past had fluoride added to drinking water.

8. Name the judge and important Scottish court case involving fluoride, and describe what is meant by the term *ultra vires*?

9. When was the *Knox report* published and what did it show?

10. List the date and conclusions of the York review.

11. What percentage of England's population now has fluoridated water?

12. List the three most beneficial ways of receiving fluoride artificially (not including water).

13. How can fluoride be administered to babies under 2 years and children from 2 to 13 years?

14. Which children should receive fluoride supplements?

15. What dose of fluoride tablet would you give to a high-risk 6-year-old when the level of fluoride in the drinking water is below 0.3 ppm?

16. What are the maximum levels of fluoride recommended in toothpastes for children under 3 years, over 3 years and for adults?

FLUORIDE

REFERENCES

1. Levine, R.S., Stillman-Lowe, C.R. (2004) *The Scientific Basis of Oral Health Education*. BDJ Books, London.
2. Collins, W.J., Walsh, T., Figures, K. (1999) *A Handbook for Dental Hygienists*, 4th edn. Butterworth Heinemann, Oxford.
3. Fejerskov, O., Kidd, E. (2004) *Dental Caries, The Disease and Its Clinical Management*. Blackwell Munksgaard, Oxford.
4. The British Fluoridation Society (1983) *Comments on the Case Mrs Catherine McColl v Strathclyde Regional Council Held in the Court of Session, Edinburgh*. The British Fluoridation Society, Department of Clinical Dental Sciences, University of Liverpool.

5. British Fluoridation Society (1985) *A Summary of the Knox Report and How It Refutes the Alleged Fluoridation – Cancer link*. The British Fluoridation Society, Department of Clinical Dental Sciences, University of Liverpool.
6. British Fluoridation Society (2005) *Water Fluoridation: A Briefing on the York University Systematic Review and Subsequent Research Developments*. The British Fluoridation Society, Department of Clinical Dental Sciences, University of Liverpool.
7. National Fluoride Information Centre (2007). Available at www.fluoride-information.com.
8. Bajaj, A. (2005) Water Fluoridation, *Vital Journal*, 2(Autumn), 37–39.

Chapter 12

Fissure sealants

LEARNING OUTCOMES

By the end of this chapter you should be able to:

1. Define a *fissure sealant*, explain why it is used and identify sites most commonly sealed and materials most commonly used in sealing.

2. Describe *fissure sealing techniques*.

3. List several trials which provide evidence for the effectiveness of fissure sealants.

WHAT IS A FISSURE SEALANT?

A *fissure sealant* is a plastic resin material placed in pits and fissures of molar teeth (less common in premolars), cingulums and palatal grooves of incisors, in order to prevent or arrest the development of caries.

Fissure sealants were first developed in the 1970s as a preventive measure. Unlike amalgam restorations, there is no preparatory cutting or drilling of the enamel surface of the tooth unless caries is present.

Reasons for using fissure sealants

Fissure sealants make teeth easier to clean and protect surfaces from plaque. Fissures in newly erupted permanent molars are too small to be penetrated by toothbrush bristles and plaque is often trapped here, leading to the development of caries[1]. Caries of first permanent molars (sixes) in 12-year-old English school children accounts for the majority of tooth decay at this age[2], and caries of the occlusal surfaces accounts for 50% of decay in first molars[3].

Enamel is not fully hardened by the time of eruption. *Maturation* (hardening) of the enamel takes several years to complete and the probability of a caries attack reaches a peak at 2–4 years post-eruption. However, maturation is more rapid in the presence of fluoride, so all children should use fluoride toothpaste to assist this process as well as to help prevent caries. Fluoride applied topically helps to strengthen enamel as well as interfere with bacterial reproduction.

When and where to seal

Fissure sealing can be carried out in older children and adults, but is most effective when placed during the early months after eruption (i.e. when the enamel is not fully mature). Fissure sealants are sometimes carried out in teenage children, as soon as the second molars (*sevens*) erupt.

Fissure sealants are most commonly used in the following cases:

- Newly erupted teeth (usually 6s and 7s) – which should be fully erupted with no flaps or contamination from saliva, which may result in failure of the sealant.
- Sticky fissures susceptible to food debris and bacteria in all children.
- Deep cingulums and buccal or palatal grooves.
- Patients susceptible to caries (family history of caries in deciduous teeth).
- Patients with a serious medical condition (e.g. congenital heart disease, haemophilia) who need to avoid dental extractions.
- Patients who are unable to cope with adequate cleaning and dental treatment.

All patients should be given further preventative advice at the same time as sealants are applied, with reference to:

- Diet (e.g. frequency of sugar, with an aim to reduce total sugar intake).
- Effective oral hygiene regimen (e.g. size of toothbrush head, frequency of toothbrushing).
- Use of fluoride.

Fissure sealant materials

Sealants are divided into two groups: *filled* and *unfilled*. Some sealants, which are filled with *lithium alumina silicate*, are more resistant to abrasion, have a prolonged life and are easier to see in the tooth[4].

There are several materials in common use; the *glass ionomer composite* (GIC) is sometimes used, but has been shown in research to be less effective than *composite resins*[5] (largely because appointment-keeping was poor).

FISSURE SEALANTS

However, glass ionomers are effective as temporary sealants in un-cooperative patients or those with partially erupted teeth and can be placed in the presence of saliva[6].

The more commonly used composite resins can be used in several ways:

- Two solutions are mixed together and polymerise by chemical reaction (rarely used).
- White light polymerised sealants. These are applied and sealed by a quartz halogen bulb, which is considered safer than plasma lights and ultraviolet lights (now considered obsolete)[6].

Sealant placement

Oral health educators (OHEs) may need to explain the sealant procedure to parents, and must therefore be familiar with the technique (although this is not the responsibility of the OHE to carry out treatment). Read the instructions on the box (and follow if different from below):

1. Polishing with a fluoride-free paste or pumice used to be advised, but this is now regarded as debatable as polish may remain deep in fissures, inhibiting retention[6].
2. Isolate the tooth with a *rubber dam* (often not tolerated well by small children) or cotton wool rolls. Dry the tooth surface with oil-free air.
3. Etch the surface of the tooth for 15–20 s with phosphoric acid (35% solution).
4. Wash the surface with an air syringe for 15 s, taking care to avoid contamination from saliva, which is the most common reason for failure of fissure sealants. If contamination occurs, re-etch and then dry the surface until it appears frosted.
5. Apply sealant, taking care that it flows across the surface in one direction (to avoid air bubbles). Remove any air bubbles carefully with a probe.
6. Polymerise using a white light for 20–30 s.
7. Check *bite* – no need to adjust as sealant wears down fairly quickly. Check interdentally with floss.

Self-etching systems are under trial but appear to give inferior retention. They should be restricted to un-cooperative patients and regarded as temporary.

Preventive resin restorations (PRR) should be used where pits and fissures are decayed. The carious area should be cleaned and filled with glass ionomer and then the non-carious area should be fissure-sealed.

It is essential to check fissure sealants regularly, and any defects in the sealant should be repaired to prevent leakage and bacterial invasion.

Tips on fissure sealing in children

Fissure sealants are the first clinical intervention in the dental chair for many children. Other children may be frightened if their first experience of dentistry has been extraction under general anaesthesia. The OHE may be able to help with calming small children and make the experience fun by explaining that:

- They will need to sit still for a couple of minutes for each tooth, with an opportunity to 'have a wriggle' between sealing teeth.
- A big, wide mouth will help the operator to see the teeth at the back.

If time permits, show children the equipment which will be used: the airwater syringe and *sealing light*, and explain the necessity for sitting very still, whilst listening for the 'bleeps'.

Clinical trials

Clinical trials, which can be used as evidence of the effectiveness of fissure sealing in preventing development of caries, have been carried out by:

- British Society for Paediatric Dentistry[7]
- Rock *et al.*[8]
- British Association for the study of Community Dentistry[9]

Remember! The names of the above trials.

FISSURE SEALANTS

SELF-ASSESSMENT

1. Define a fissure sealant and state where in the tooth it is commonly used.
2. Which materials are most often used in fissure sealing?
3. When are glass ionomer composites (GICs) used, and why?
4. Which teeth are usually sealed and at what approximate ages?
5. List six cases in which fissure sealing would be advisable.
6. What oral health advice would you give a parent and child before fissure sealing?

7. List the stages in fissure sealant placement. How would you enlist the child's full cooperation?

8. List three trials associated with the effectiveness of fissure sealing.

REFERENCES

1. Wrigley (2006) *Advice on Pit and Fissure Sealants*, Handout 19, Wrigley Oral Healthcare in Action. Available at www.betteroralhealth.info.

2. Office for National Statistics (2004) *2003 Dental Health Survey of Children and Young People*. Stationery Office Books, London.

3. Welbury, R., Raadal, M., Lygidakis, N. (2004) *Guidelines on the Use of Pit and Fissures Sealants in Paediatric Dentistry: An EAPD Policy Document*, European Academy of Paediatric Dentistry. Available at http://www.eapd.gr/EAPDJournal.

4. Collins, W.J., Walsh, T., Figures, K. (1999) *A Handbook for Dental Hygienists*, 4th edn. Butterworth Heinemann, Oxford.

5. Chadwick, B. (2005) *A randomised controlled trial to determine the effectiveness of glass ionomer sealants in pre-school children*, Caries Research, 39(1), 34–40.

6. Deery, C. (January 2007) Fissure sealants: an update and future trends, *Dental Health Journal*, 46(1), 5–9.

7. British Association for Study of Paediatric Dentistry (November 2006) A randomised controlled trial of the effectiveness of a one-step conditioning agent in sealant placement: 6 month results, *International Journal of Paediatric Dentistry*, 16(6), 424.

8. Rock, W.P., Evans, R.I.W. (1983) A comparative study between chemically polymerized fissure sealant and a light-cured resin, *British Dental Journal*, 155(10), 344–346.

9. Pitts, N.B., Evans, D.J., Nugent, Z.J. (1996) The dental caries experience of 14-year-old children in the United Kingdom. Surveys coordinated by the British Association for the Study of Community Dentistry in 1994/1995, *Community Dental Health*, 13(1), 51–58.

FISSURE SEALANTS

Chapter 13
Smoking cessation

LEARNING OUTCOMES

By the end of this chapter you should be able to:

1. List reasons why people smoke.

2. List common types of nicotine replacement therapy products available.

3. Explain the effects of smoking on the general health of adults, children and the foetus.

4. List smoking-related conditions.

5. Describe the *Process of Change* and draw Prochaska and DiClemente's *Cycle of Change*.

INTRODUCTION

Dental professionals have long been aware of the damaging effects of tobacco smoking upon oral as well as general health. However, they are often surprised to find that many patients still have little knowledge of the effects of smoking on their oral tissues.

One of the ways in which oral health educators (OHEs) can improve oral and general health is by educating and encouraging patients to stop smoking. Patients will only change their behaviour if they have the knowledge to do so and their attitude is geared towards a behavioural change.

REASONS WHY PEOPLE SMOKE

Many people who smoke want to stop. They have the knowledge about why they should give up, but not the willpower to do so and require a change in attitude.

Attitudes are formed from personal experiences throughout life and encompass influences from family and friends, values and beliefs. Patients must have a strong desire to change their behaviour before they will do so. In order to influence them to stop smoking, the OHE needs to have some knowledge of the reasons why people smoke:

- It makes them feel grown up amongst their peers (pre-teens/younger teenagers).

- They began smoking before the dangers were recognised, enjoy it and see no reason to stop (older people).

- To relieve stress (even though nicotine is actually a stimulant). This is the most common reason the OHE will be given, and the usual reason for a relapse.

- To keep weight down. A particularly important reason given by women.

- Social reasons. They may have the odd cigarette on an evening out – but are not addicted.

- They are addicted. Many people in this group want to change their behaviour, yet cannot break the habit.

EFFECTS OF TOBACCO SMOKING ON GENERAL HEALTH

The OHE also needs to know the potential effects of tobacco smoking on general health, in order to help change patients' attitudes. Conditions and consequences include:

- Chronic bronchitis

- Emphysema

- Coronary artery disease

- Peripheral vascular disease (can lead to impotence)

- Infertility

- Certain cancers, particularly of the lung, mouth, larynx, oesophagus and bladder. The combined effects of smoking and moderate–high alcohol consumption (particularly spirits) increases the likelihood of cancer.

- Increased risk of miscarriage, premature labour, prenatal death, low birth weight and reduced educational attainment of a child. Research[1] has shown that children of mothers who smoke during pregnancy have a higher caries rate.

- Passive smoking is especially dangerous in children and can cause sudden infant death syndrome, respiratory infections, asthma, 'glue ear', short stature, hospital admission and school absenteeism.

EFFECTS OF TOBACCO SMOKING ON ORAL HEALTH

Effects on the oral health include:

- Stickier plaque
- Stained teeth
- Halitosis
- Xerostomia
- Hairy tongue
- Loss of taste (and smell)
- Destruction of the periodontium
- Increased risk of oral cancer

HELPING PATIENTS CHANGE SMOKING HABITS

Patients may ask OHEs for help, and the OHE may be able to help motivate them towards change. However, the OHE is unlikely to change the behaviour of someone who has not made a decision to stop smoking. Patients in the UK should seek help from a trained smoking cessation advisor (available at some doctors' surgeries), or NHS specialist services.

The process of change

By studying the theory of changing behaviour, the OHE will have a better knowledge on the stages people go through when quitting.

In 1986, two educators called *Prochaska* and *DiClemente* developed a theory called the *Process of Change*[2]. They believed that changing attitudes and behaviour is a continuous cycle, rather than a single occurrence. Their theories

SMOKING CESSATION

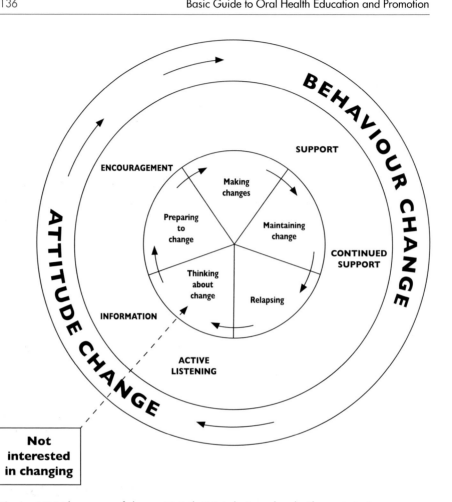

Figure 13.1 The process of change (© Ruth McIntosh. Reproduced with permission)

can be applied to many circumstances, smoking cessation being just one example. Many patients regard stopping their habit as a one-off event and see the resumption of the habit as failure. The OHE's role is to help patients see it as a continual process (Figure 13.1).

The stages of the cycle and an example of each stage (related in this case to smoking) are shown in italics.

1. Thinking about change
   Concerned smoker – worried about the effects of smoking or thinking of quitting.

2. Preparing to change
   Planning to quit – getting ready to quit – setting a quit date.

3. Making the change
   Action (quit day) – actually stopping smoking.

4. Maintaining the change
   Maintain a quit attempt – resisting relapse.

5. Relapse
   Has gone back to smoking – could be temporary or long term.

The important thing for the OHE to stress is that a relapse is not the end of the cycle, but the part which precedes beginning again. Be prepared to spend time listening, talking and empathising with patients, but never try to sound judgemental or patronising; some smokers are *contented* and not interested in quitting. The OHE will encounter resentment if they apply pressure for change.

Patients who decide to stop will need:

- Empathy (includes active listening).

- Understanding (includes giving accurate information or signposting appropriately).

- Encouragement (it helps to know that your dentist and staff really care).

- Support (often over a long period). Patients need to know that they can come back to the OHE when their resolve weakens, or life events increase their stress.

Remember! The OHE should ask for help from people with more experience if feeling 'out of their depth' when advising patients who want to stop smoking.

Nicotine replacement therapy

The chances of smoking cessation for many patients increase when nicotine addiction is managed alongside a change in behaviour. Pharmacological support in the form of nicotine replacement therapy (NRT), should be considered.

There are different ways of delivering NRT to meet nicotine withdrawal symptoms. Products include adhesive patches, nasal sprays, inhalators (look like cigarettes), chewing gum, lozenges and micro-tabs (placed under the tongue). The choice of which NRT product to use is made after discussing and evaluating an individual's smoking habit. It is common to use a patch and an oral product together. (Zyban® and Champix® are not NRT, but drugs which work on altering chemical messages in the brain, and should only be used on medical advice from a doctor.)

SMOKING CESSATION

Champix® (a trade name for verenicline) was first licensed in the UK in December 2006. It mimics the effect of nicotine on the body (by stimulating brain receptors), reduces smoking urges and relieves withdrawal symptoms. It also partially blocks receptors and prevents nicotine from attaching to them to help those who give in to temptation.

SELF-ASSESSMENT

1. List reasons people give for smoking.

2. List general and oral health conditions commonly associated with smoking in smokers and those close to them (i.e. children and unborn babies).

3. Briefly explain Prochaska and DiClemente's *Process of Change*. Draw the circular diagram illustrating this.

4. Write a paragraph explaining how you as an OHE could help support a smoker thinking about making a quit attempt, mentioning the therapies available.

REFERENCES

1. Haiek, P. (2006) *Smoking Cessation Training and Research Programme (Maudsley Clinic Model)*. Park Crescent Conference Centre, London, 3–5 July 2006.
2. Ireland, R. (2004) *Advanced Dental Nursing*. Blackwell Science Ltd., Oxford.

SMOKING CESSATION

SECTION 4
DELIVERING ORAL HEALTH MESSAGES

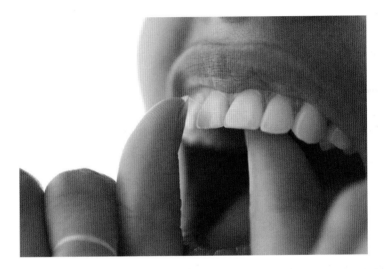

INTRODUCTION

This section is concerned with delivering the messages learned in the preceding sections, including effective toothbrushing, reducing sugars in the diet, the use of fluoride and preventive treatment such as fissure sealing.

It examines the oral health educator's (OHE's) role as a communicator, and provides general knowledge of the basic principles of education and educational theories (ideas of eminent educators upon whose doctrines educational principles have been established). Modern-day influences of the media and the use of information technology in teaching and producing resources are also discussed.

There is advice on setting up a preventive dental unit, obtaining or making resources for use in delivering messages, and how to prepare for oral hygiene sessions and exhibitions in or outside the workplace. Delivering information on anti-plaque agents and practical oral hygiene instruction are also addressed.

Chapter 14
Communication

LEARNING OUTCOMES

By the end of this chapter you should be able to:

1. Define *communication*.
2. List and briefly describe the three main aspects of *effective communication*.
3. Recognise communication barriers.
4. Quote the *three rules of communication*.
5. Recognise the increasing role of the media in communicating with the public.
6. Outline the use of information technology by the OHE.
7. Define *information fade*.

WHAT IS COMMUNICATION?

Communication involves the sending of a message by one individual and the receiving of the same message by another individual.

Communication is what oral health education is all about. Being able to communicate a message to a variety of patients (some of whom want to hear it, and others who do not) is tantamount to success for the OHE.

Most patients will have experienced occasions on leaving the surgery of a doctor, dentist or other health professional feeling annoyed, confused or even more nervous than when they arrived. The onus to put the patient at ease, answer questions truthfully and explain points clearly and concisely lies with the professional. It is not the patient's fault if a message is not understood. It is therefore important for the OHE to know a little communication theory.

COMMUNICATION IN THE DENTAL SURGERY

As mentioned, the responsibility for good communication lies with the professional and forms the basis of a good relationship between a dental professional and a patient.

Communication takes place at two levels (E. Hill, personal communications):

1. Cognitive (understanding)

2. Emotional (related to feelings)

In a dental situation, the latter is often more important.

Effective communication

Effective communication makes it easier for patients to discuss problems and devise solutions.

Three main aspects of effective (or *facilitative*) communication that the OHE should practise are warmth, empathy and respect.

Warmth

Warmth demonstrates interest and concern for the patient. Warmth is communicated primarily through non-verbal behaviour, such as:

- Eye contact (particularly important)
- Head-nodding
- Facial expressions
- Other non-verbal signs of interest and attention

Empathy

Empathy means perceiving and understanding a situation from the viewpoint of another. For the OHE, it is the most important characteristic of facilitative communication. Empathy conveys the message: 'I care enough to try to understand your feelings and point of view'.

Respect

Respect is an awareness that others are entitled to have feelings and perceptions different from those of the professional. It does not necessarily imply agreement.

COMMUNICATION

Communication barriers

Recognising that barriers exist is the first stage in establishing communication in the surgery. The following barriers have been identified (F. Marriott, personal communications).

Social/cultural barriers

There may be a social or cultural gap between the educator and patient. Barriers include:

- Ethnic background
- Social class (identified by dress, language, accent)
- Cultural/religious beliefs (e.g. hygiene, nutrition)
- Values
- Age/sex

Limited receptiveness of patient

The OHE may want to communicate with the patient but not the reverse. Certain patients may be unreceptive to the health professional for reasons including:

- Mental health problems or confusion
- Illness, tiredness or pain
- Emotional distress or fear
- Busy or distracted
- Low self-esteem (not valuing themselves or their health)

Negative attitude towards the OHE

Some patients may be *anti* the educator even before they have met because:

- Of a previous bad experience.
- They never trust people in authority.
- They see the educator as a threat (someone who will criticise or judge).
- An OHE's example conflicts with advice (e.g. educator with halitosis).

COMMUNICATION

- The patient believes they know it *all* already.
- Patient has a subconscious wish not to know (e.g. results of medical tests).

Limited understanding or poor memory

Patients may have difficulties because:

- Of a limited intelligence/lack of education/illiteracy
- Their understanding of language may be poor
- OHE uses jargon
- Poor memory (cannot remember advice)

Insufficient emphasis on education by professional

Communication may fail because the professional does not give sufficient time or attention to improving skills. This may be because:

- It was given a low priority in basic training
- It is discouraged/given low priority in the practice
- Of a lack of confidence in own skills and knowledge
- Inadequate training/failure to keep up to date
- Hurried approach (not enough time allowed)

Contradictory messages

Confusion arises when patients receive different messages from other health professionals, such as:

- Dentists
- Doctors and health visitors
- Well-meaning family and friends
- Experts 'change their minds' as knowledge improves

Remember! Barriers to effective communication can lead to 'information fade'. It has been shown that patients only remember 10% of the information given by the dental professional (M. Midda, personal communications). It is therefore useful to reinforce the information given by giving the patient a leaflet to take away. Leaflets on many topics can be obtained from the representatives of dental companies or from health promotion units found in larger towns and cities in the UK, or OHEs can design their own.

MEDIA INFLUENCE

It is increasingly apparent that the public is greatly influenced by advertising campaigns in publications and on television. Patients will ask OHEs about the merits of different oral health products seen and heard about. It is important that the OHEs listen to their views and show no bias, and remain abreast of current media articles and information, whilst remaining aware that there may not be an evidence base for the claims made (F. Marriott, personal communications).

OHEs should therefore read dental journals and publications on a regular basis (sometimes reading articles can be documented and put down as continuing professional development in the UK).

TECHNOLOGY AND THE OHE

Computers are playing an increasing part in day-to-day activities and it is inevitable that health professionals giving oral health education are making more and more use of them. In most dental surgeries, record keeping has been simplified by the installation of computers. Printers, DVD players, fax machines and mobile telephones are also important facilitators in communication between dental staff and patients.

Technology in the surgery or PDU

Technology may be of use to the OHE in the following ways:

- Making appointments.

- Storing records of work done with patients on each visit – so information is easily accessible, and easy to see if agreed targets have been achieved.

- Communication using CD-ROM, DVDs and videos. Many surgeries now have media players in the waiting room or a PDU so that patients can be left to view information.

- The Internet is an excellent source of oral health information for OHEs and their patients.

COMMUNICATION

Technology and OHE resources

Computers, the Internet and other technological advances have also revolutionised the way resources and projects have been produced by OHE students. It is now possible to produce resource material of a very high standard for use with patients, including:

- Displays for use in exhibitions

- Laminated backup leaflets for patients

- Laminated posters

- Digital photographs

Remember! The three rules of communication:

Tell me. . . . . I forget

Show me. . . . . I remember

Involve me. . . . . I learn

Care about your patients, be nice to them and they will do anything that is asked of them.

SELF-ASSESSMENT

1. Define *communication.*

2. Name two levels of communication.

3. Name the three qualities needed by the OHE in order to facilitate communication.

4. List six possible barriers to communication.

5. List the *three rules of communication.*

6. Write short notes on how *effective communication* can be established between an OHE and a patient on a one-to-one basis. What factors may prevent effective communication?

7. How should the OHE deal with patients who are uncertain about the use of products promoted by the media?

COMMUNICATION

Chapter 15
Principles of education

LEARNING OUTCOMES

By the end of this chapter you should be able to:

1. List and briefly describe the *three domains of learning*.

2. Explain the difference between *aims* and *objectives*.

3. Write aims and objectives for a teaching session.

4. Construct a lesson plan and questionnaire.

5. Answer written questions on *evaluation*.

INTRODUCTION

When educating a patient, oral health educators (OHEs) pass on expertise and their own feelings about what is being taught. The patient absorbs the information and acquires new knowledge, skills and attitudes.

Teaching does not just 'happen', and has to be learned and planned meticulously. Before OHEs can teach or pass on knowledge, they need the basic skills to do so. These skills are known as the *principles of education*.

EDUCATIONAL THEORISTS

Education is based on theories formulated over many years by eminent academics, and the OHE should be aware of the theories of Tones and Tannahill (two expert educationalists).

Tones's *Model for Health Promotion* (1993)[1] emphasised that illness is not the responsibility of the individual alone, and that many factors contribute to it, including social and environmental circumstances.

Another theorist called Tannahill produced a model of health promotion concerned with three main areas[2]:

- Health education – educating children in healthy lifestyles.

- Health prevention – detecting problems such as smoking or alcohol abuse.

- Heath protection – government legislation in protecting the public (e.g. drink-driving laws and more recently smoking bans in public places).

Education experts have proved that individuals absorb what they are taught in ways related to previous experiences[3].

THE THREE DOMAINS OF LEARNING

Blinkhorn[4] described in detail how people learn in three different ways, known as the *domains of learning*. Before structuring a session, the OHE must decide upon which domain their session falls into:

1. Knowledge-related (*cognitive*). Receiving new information or explanations and thus increasing knowledge (e.g. explaining what causes caries).

2. Attitude-related. Forming and changing attitudes, beliefs, values and opinions (e.g. a nervous patient being persuaded to visit the dentist).

3. Behaviour-related. Acquiring and improving skills (e.g. toothbrushing).

Remember! *KAB*: Knowledge, Attitudes, Behaviour.

STRUCTURING A LESSON

After considering which domain of learning a teaching session is concerned with, the OHE is ready to proceed with structuring a lesson.

However brief a session with a patient, it is important that it is planned and structured. (Whilst the *patient* is referred to throughout this chapter, the information is equally applicable when teaching groups.)

As well as setting aims and objectives, the educator should construct and follow a lesson plan, and devise an evaluation process (to gauge how successful elements of the lesson were):

- Aims and objectives – education begins with a goal (an *aim*), and the means of achieving that goal (*objectives*).
- A lesson plan – detailed chronologically.
- Evaluation – to gauge how successful elements of the lesson were.

Aims

An *aim* is a goal or an intention to achieve something, and is quite often general and non-specific. It should detail what the patient needs to know. Aims should be:

- Brief
- Clear
- Simple
- Comprehensive (covering all the material to be taught in a session)

For example: 'I aim to teach this patient how to brush effectively'.

Objectives

After stating the intention of the session, the next step is to plan how to achieve it.

Objectives state what the patient will be able to achieve at the end of a session. Objectives should be[4]:

- Specific (state exactly what the patient will achieve).
- Measurable (there will be a means of testing new skills, knowledge or attitude).
- Attainable (the learning ability of the patient must be considered).
- Relevant (relating to what you want the patient to achieve).
- Time-related (what is achievable in the time available).

Remember! SMART
For example: by the end of the session a patient will be able to:

- Select a suitable toothbrush for their needs.
- Carry out efficient brushing techniques.

PRINCIPLES OF EDUCATION

When setting objectives, the OHE must first consider:

- The age, sex and social class of the patient.
- Previous knowledge and attitudes.
- Resources available.
- Time allocated for the session.
- What the patient should realistically be able to achieve after the session.

Words such as *know*, *understand* and *feel* should be avoided because they are not measurable. The OHE needs *measurable objectives*, using words such as *explain*, *describe*, *state*, *demonstrate* and *discuss*.

Remember! An *aim* is a statement of intent, purpose or a goal. *Objectives* are statements of what a patient will be able to achieve after a session.

Once it is known *what* to teach, the educator must plan *how* to achieve these goals using a lesson plan.

Lesson plan

All lessons, no matter how short, need a plan. A plan enables the educator to:

- Keep to the topic
- Refer to objectives
- Keep to the teaching method
- Keep to timescales
- Assess how well the patient learned
- Evaluate the lesson

It is recommended that a lesson plan comprises a table (e.g. Table 15.1), or a logical list of topics to cover.

As educators gain experience, they will refer to plans less and less. However, it is still a good idea to have a plan to double-check that nothing has been forgotten.

Teaching methods

This book does cover teaching methods in detail, but OHEs should be aware that there are many methods, and that not all patients respond to the same

Table 15.1 Example lesson plan – principles of education

Timing	Objectives	Subject	Method	Resources	Evaluation method
10.00 am	Introduction	Principles of education	Talk	N/A	Body language
10.05 am	Objective 1	Three domains of leaning	PowerPoint® presentation	Computer equipment	Questions and answers
10.15 am	Objective 2	Aims and objectives	As above	As above	As above
10.35 am	Objective 3	Writing aims and objectives	Student participation	Pens, paper	Verbal feedback
10.50 am	Objective 4	Construct a lesson plan	Group planning	Pens, blank lesson plans	Tutor feedback
11.05 am	Objective 5	Evaluation	PowerPoint® presentation	Computer equipment	Answer written questions
11.25 am	Objective 6	Closing remarks	Talk	N/A	NA
11.30 am	Finish				

approach. For example: some patients like to demonstrate what they have learned back to you, others will not, and certain patients remember better if points are written down for them. Experience will gradually help the OHE plan and vary methods of teaching accordingly.

Evaluation

Each teaching session needs to be *evaluated*.

In the context of oral health education, the term *evaluation* is used to quantify to what extent advice given to the patient produces tangible results. It can be defined as: 'making a judgement about the outcome and effectiveness of an oral health education session or programme'.

Effective evaluation will tell you:

- Whether objectives have been achieved
- If the educator's efforts were worthwhile

Evaluation types

Before deciding upon an evaluation method, it is worth exploring different types of evaluation in order to select the most appropriate for a teaching session.

Outcome evaluation

What will be the outcome of the session? Will patients increase their knowledge, or change their behaviour or attitude as a result? (**Remember!** *KAB.*)

Process evaluation

This is concerned with session delivery as it happens. Is the teaching process going well? This can usually be surmised by patients' reactions, or the signals they are giving. Do they look interested and attentive, or are they fidgeting and looking out of the window? From learning to spot the signs, it is possible to continually *process evaluate* and adapt a session.

Patient evaluation

What are patients telling you? Observe non-verbal feedback: facial expressions and body language. Take on feedback and be prepared to modify your teaching in future sessions.

Peer evaluation

Feedback from colleagues. Ask for comments and suggestions to improve future sessions.

Self-evaluation (reflective practice)

Look at your performance after a session. How well did it go? What did not work and why? How could the session be improved? It is a good idea to keep a *reflective practice* notebook, jotting down notes about what happened immediately after each session. This enables you to identify problems and improve performance.

Evaluation methods

Having identified suitable evaluation types, the OHE must then select which evaluation methods to employ. In other words, how to assess how well a teaching session worked.

There are many methods, but whichever one is chosen, bear in mind that it must relate back to aims and objectives, and show whether the goals were achieved or not.

Evaluation methods include:

- *Question and answer* session with patient – skilful questioning will help patients give full, clear, honest answers.

- Patient demonstration of new skill – *visual evaluation*.

- Records of behaviour change – (e.g. plaque scores, indices, documented decrease in caries rate). Help from the dentist or hygienist may be required here.

- Questionnaire. This has the disadvantage in that patients will often give the answer they think the educator is expecting, rather than what they really believe. Designing an effective questionnaire is complex and requires skill and experience.

SO WHAT IS A QUESTIONNAIRE?

A questionnaire is a relatively inexpensive and swift mechanism for collecting information or data that can be easily analysed and interpreted.

To produce a successful questionnaire the OHE will need:

- A clear idea of an overall goal (aims and objectives).

- A good knowledge of the subject.

PRINCIPLES OF EDUCATION

- Background information on the target group (what do they know?).

- To decide upon exactly what information needs to be answered (using *open* and *closed* questions).

Open and closed questions

There are two main types of questions in a questionnaire:

- *Open Questions* – which provide qualitative data. For example: 'What kind of toothbrush will you use now that you have seen my exhibition?'

- *Closed questions* – which provide *quantitative* data. For example: 'Will you now use a smaller-headed toothbrush?'

Advantages of open questions:

- Respondent can use own words to reply (e.g. 'I will use a small-headed, medium, nylon brush').

- Good when used in a *pilot study*; useful for finding out what people know and do not know, and can help the phrasing of questions in the final questionnaire accordingly.

Disadvantages of open questions:

- Analysis is more difficult and time-consuming to measure than *closed questions*.

Advantages of closed questions:

- Quick to complete – respondents just tick 'Yes' or 'No'.

- Easy analysis – questioner counts 'Yes' or 'No' answers.

Disadvantages of closed questions:

- May result in leading questions (i.e. respondents may answer as to what they think you wish to know).

- Loss of depth – does not find out people's opinions.

Whether the educator decides to use open or closed questions (or both), care should be taken to avoid questions that are:

- Irrelevant – do not tell you what you want to know

- Offensive – make respondents feel small or embarrassed

- Ambiguous – can be interpreted in more than one way

It is good practice to allow respondents to remain anonymous should they wish, and a choice of 'opting out' of answering any question they may not be comfortable with. Confidentiality is also an important consideration.

Once the type of questions has been decided upon, the next stage is to design the questionnaire.

Questionnaire design

When designing a questionnaire take into account the following considerations:

- Will a brief pilot questionnaire with a few respondents be helpful?

- Decide how many questions are required (10 or less if possible – people get bored and mind-boggled if there are too many).

- Refer back to aims and objectives to clarify the direction.

- Write questions in easy-to-understand language.

- Give clear instructions on how to answer (e.g. 'Please tick or circle either Yes or No')

- If using open questions, leave sufficient space for writing answers.

- Plan how and when questionnaires will be handed out.

- Think about how they will be collected (easy if you are there when they are completed, but notoriously difficult if people take them home – you will be lucky to see them again).

- Consider costs (e.g. postage).

SELF-ASSESSMENT

1. Write aims and objectives for the following lesson: 'You have been asked to improve the toothbrushing skills for a mixed class of twenty 10-year-olds in a classroom setting'.

2. What is meant by the *evaluation* of an oral health session?

3. Briefly discuss the methods available for evaluating the outcomes of an OHE session.

4. What is meant by the term reflective practice? How is this achieved before, during, and after a dental health session?

5. Design a questionnaire:

   – Choose a topic that interests you and is relevant to your workplace, and identify your target group.

   – Write *aims and objectives*, and eight questions based on the objectives.

   – Begin with a brief explanation to participants. For example: 'Please complete the following questionnaire to help me with my Dental Health Exhibition. Read the questions and tick or circle the appropriate answer'.

   – At the end of your questionnaire you can write something like 'Thank you for answering my questionnaire. Please place your completed copy in the box to the right of my display'.

REFERENCES

1. Wilson-Barnett, J. (2 April 2002) The theory of health promotion: implications for nursing, *Nursing Times*, 98(14), 43.
2. Sunderland University. Available at www.sunderland.ac.uk.
3. Reece, I., Walker, S. (1992) *A Practical Guide to Teaching, Training, Learning*, Business Education Publishers Ltd., Sunderland.
4. Blinkhorn, A.S. (2001) *Notes on Oral Health*, 5th edn. Eden Bianchi Press, Manchester.

PRINCIPLES OF EDUCATION

Chapter 16

Setting up a preventive dental unit (PDU)

LEARNING OUTCOMES

By the end of this chapter you should be able to:

1. Describe the characteristics of a well-organised PDU.

2. Explain the factors to be considered in setting up a PDU.

3. List the points to remember when organising a display.

INTRODUCTION

A PDU (Figure 16.1) is ideally a self-contained area where oral health education can be given to individuals or small groups without interruption from the dental surgery. In some surgeries, there is no space for a separate PDU, but an enthusiastic educator will be able to find ways around this and adapt existing facilities.

In setting up a PDU you will need:

- A business plan/marketing strategy

- Enthusiasm/support from employers

- A viable and flexible budget

- A suitable location

- Well-trained staff (motivated and communicative)

The PDU is an area which is used to motivate and communicate with patients, often establishing a friendly, informal relationship that is not always possible during routine dental treatment. Successful preventative treatment is dependent on patient and staff cooperation, and it is wise to consult the dental

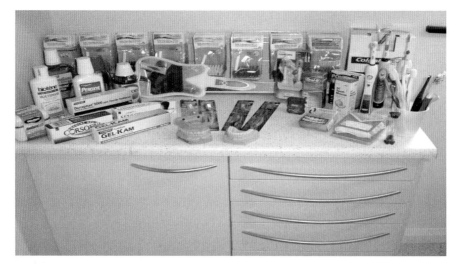

Figure 16.1 A preventative dental unit (PDU) (© Elizabeth Hill. Reproduced with permission)

team (a short questionnaire could be used to ascertain the dental team's ideas). Another consideration when setting up a PDU is to take into account the practice catchment area, i.e. whether it is situated in:

- A city-centre location
- A rural area
- A suburban area
- An industrial area
- An ethnic minority area

Time and resources will need to be adapted according to the location of your PDU. For example: people attending a city centre practice will probably appreciate dinner-hour appointments. People in a rural area may have more time but may rely on infrequent buses for transport. All these points need to be considered and discussed with your colleagues. Regular staff meetings are important to keep staff motivation up and to provide/receive feedback from staff (E. Hill, personal communications).

PDU LOCATION

Here are some suggestions:

- A spare room

SETTING UP A PREVENTIVE
DENTAL UNIT (PDU)

- A partitioned area

- An adapted corner of a dental surgery or other clinical area

- The waiting room (outside of surgery hours)

Where space is very limited, portable PDU display cabinets (which fold away for storage) can be obtained from certain dental suppliers (P. Riley, personal communications).

PDU DESIGN

The PDU should ideally be a place in which patients can feel relaxed and are able to discuss dental problems. If possible, it should be separate from the surgery (non-clinical and non-threatening), as patients are often put off by surgery sounds/smells.

Decor should take into account different age groups, and so it should include areas suitable for motivating adults, teenagers and small children.

A well-designed PDU should have the following attributes:

- Good lighting

- Easy access (elderly/disabled)

- Soft, hardwearing floor (children will be sitting here to play)

- Robust fittings/furniture

- Easily-cleaned worktops – varying heights appropriate to target groups

- Space for displays

- Sink(s)

- Large, well-lit mirror(s)

- Motivational aids (well-displayed)

- Appropriate toys (e.g. play foods, books about visiting dentist)

SETTING UP DISPLAYS

Display boards can be obtained from office equipment suppliers, or sometimes 'begged' from refurbishing offices or department stores. Make full use of wall

SETTING UP A PREVENTIVE DENTAL UNIT (PDU)

space and worktops, bearing in mind the height of the target group (e.g. are the patients children or in wheelchairs?).

Your display may include:

- Posters (home-made or commercial) – change regularly as they soon become 'tatty'. If possible, laminate them to prevent this. When making posters, remember to keep them simple, eye-catching and clear.

- Books – there are some good books about dental visits for children.

- Toys/games appropriate to dental teaching – home-made or shop-bought 'food' toys.

- Mouth models – there are many different types on the market.

- Leaflets (home-made, using the FOG[1]/SMOG[2] indices. FOG stands for frequency of gobbledegook; SMOG stands for simple measure of gobbledegook.

- Commercial leaflets about diet or dental topics, which are frequently updated, can often be obtained from health promotion centres.

- Toothbrushes and other oral hygiene aids – commercial companies are often generous in supplying these if the practice sells their products.

ORGANISATION

This is where help and cooperation from other staff (particularly *reception*) is important.

The oral health educator (OHE) will need:

- Patient referrals – from the dentist or other health professionals.

- A well-organised appointment system, including an appointment book. Consider the length of appointments, a recall system (to keep up motivation and encourage feedback) and a facility to refer patients back to the dental surgeon/hygienist or on to a specialist.

- Flexible opening times – after school, school holidays and Saturday mornings are popular. Remember that young children have short attention spans.

- Keep to time – adults have many demands on their time.

- Evaluation procedures – use patient feedback to assess how well a PDU is working. Set up a system, such as coloured stickers on record cards, so that dentists/health professionals know who has been seen in the PDU and can therefore monitor patient progress.

SETTING UP A PREVENTIVE DENTAL UNIT (PDU)

Setting up and running a successful PDU is an interesting and rewarding challenge. Many patients, especially children, will look forward to regular appointments and dental health should improve as a result. With enthusiastic support from employers, OHEs can set up projects from time to time in the PDU. These can be very informative (covering different topics) and utilise oral health training to the full.

Now that you have the ability to set up a PDU, you can think about planning oral hygiene sessions. These may take place within your PDU or at another venue.

SELF-ASSESSMENT

1. Describe the characteristics of a well-organised PDU.

2. Explain the factors to be considered in setting up a PDU.

3. List the points to remember when organising a display.

REFERENCES

1. Blinkhorn, A.S. (2001) *Notes on Oral Health*, 5th edn. Eden Bianchi Press, Manchester.
2. Reece, I., Walker, S. (1992) *A Practical Guide to Teaching Training and Learning*, Business Education Publishers Limited, Sunderland.

SETTING UP A PREVENTIVE DENTAL UNIT (PDU)

Chapter 17

Planning an oral hygiene session

LEARNING OUTCOMES

By the end of this chapter, you should be able to:

1. List the stages in planning an oral hygiene session.
2. List the points to consider before delivering a session.
3. Write brief notes on planning a talk to a group outside of the workplace.
4. Briefly describe points to consider when setting up an exhibition.

INTRODUCTION

Careful preparation for a teaching session is essential for its success. Whether a teaching session is aimed at an individual or small or large group, the following stages in preparation are applicable:

1. Obtain background information about the target group or person you will be teaching.
2. Decide upon the topic.
3. Write aims and objectives.
4. Select visual aids and other resources.
5. Plan assessment and evaluation.
6. Create a lesson plan.
7. Rehearse (if possible).

Points to consider when planning your oral hygiene session

When planning an oral hygiene session, the OHE should take into consideration the following points (K. Needs, J. Postans, personal communications):

- Venue (if not in a PDU) – location, access, size of room, facilities available.
- Size of group – if too big, individual attention cannot be given.
- Prior knowledge – of the group or individual.
- Subject relevance – is the topic meeting their needs?
- Timing – too long a session leads to boredom or distraction.
- Special needs – (e.g. physical or mental disabilities of patients).
- Learning abilities – high intelligence/slow learners.
- Minority ethnic groups/language barriers – will you be understood?
- Social class – bear in mind what learners can afford to buy.
- Resources/motivational aids – should be relevant and not too complex.
- Cost – keep within a specified budget.

Planning a talk to a group outside of the practice

When planning a talk outside of the practice to a group of people, the OHE should:

1. Visit the venue in advance. On a preliminary visit check:
   - Car parking/disabled access.
   - Position of the room – is it upstairs?
   - Size of room – will it be big enough, or too big?
   - Lighting/electric plugs – for using a DVD or overhead projector.
   - Fixtures and fittings – are there chairs, sinks, mirrors?
   - Resources available (e.g. TV, overhead projector, flipcharts).
2. Book a date with the venue owner or organiser (obtain proof of booking where applicable), and confirm the booking near the time.
3. Obtain background information from teacher or group leader.
4. Work out costs.
5. Decide upon aims/objectives and evaluation.

6. Collect visual aids/resources. These may include tooth and mouth cleaning aids, leaflets, posters, videos and mouth models.

7. Rehearse if possible – maybe using colleagues as an audience.

Delivering the talk (checklist)

On the actual day of the talk:

1. Check you have everything before leaving for the venue.

2. Arrive early.

3. Ensure the room is arranged as required.

4. Set out resources.

5. Welcome the audience/target group.

6. Introduce yourself and anyone else involved in delivering the session.

7. Speak slowly and clearly so that everyone can hear – ask them!

8. Encourage group participation.

9. Use a variety of teaching methods (to avoid boredom).

10. Avoid technical jargon (unless talking to fellow professionals).

11. Encourage motivation and awareness.

12. Allow supervised practice of new skills (if applicable).

13. Reinforce learning – using handouts and/or leaflets.

14. Arrange a return visit to follow up learning (if possible).

15. Finish on time – people get restless if a session overruns.

Remember to thank the target group for their attention, teachers or group leaders for their help and colleagues for support. Leave the venue as it was and send thank you letters to those involved promptly.

Setting up an exhibition

Planning an exhibition or a display also requires much thought and preparation, and the following stages should be followed:

1. Decide upon the type of exhibition (notice boards, free-standing).

2. Consider lighting and the position of the exhibition – maximise its visibility.

3. Consider the height of those who will view it.

4. Set up tables if needed.

5. Make the exhibition simple, eye-catching and interesting.

6. Organise information in short sections under clear headings.

7. Arrange times to stay with the exhibition and talk to the public/patients.

8. Prepare and supervise an evaluation method, such as pre- and post-questionnaires.

Poster design and displaying written information

When planning and preparing a poster (or other written information) for an exhibition or display, the following points should be considered:

1. Experiment with colour combinations (e.g. yellow on black shows up well; yellow on white is not good, red is eye-catching, but too much red may be overpowering).

2. Write clearly and large enough for the information to be read easily (thick felt-tip pens work well).

3. Vary the colour and size of text for extra emphasis.

4. Use different shapes and backgrounds.

Remember! Whether planning a talk or an exhibition within the practice or at an outside venue, involve colleagues whenever possible; they often have hidden talents and good ideas.

SELF-ASSESSMENT

1. List the stages involved in planning an oral health session.

2. List the points to consider before delivering a session.

3. Write brief notes on the planning stages of delivering a talk to a group outside of the practice.

4. Briefly describe how to plan and set up an exhibition or display.

PLANNING AN ORAL HYGIENE SESSION

Chapter 18
Anti-plaque agents

LEARNING OUTCOMES

By the end of this chapter you should be able to:

1. Define an anti-plaque agent, and discuss the advantages and disadvantages of using various anti-plaque aids with patients.
2. State the functions of toothpaste (containing fluoride).
3. State the percentages of the active ingredients, dosage, recommended usage and side effects of *chlorhexidine gluconate* and fluoride mouthwashes.
4. Explain when hydrogen peroxide mouthwash should be recommended.
5. List the functions of sugar-free chewing gum.

WHAT ARE ANTI-PLAQUE AGENTS?

One of the largest growth industries in the consumer market over the last two decades has been oral hygiene aids (particularly, toothpastes, mouthwashes and chewing gum).

In view of the role of bacterial plaque in periodontal disease, clinicians and manufacturers have been interested in the potential value of anti-plaque or antibacterial agents in both toothpastes and mouthwashes, and there are now so many on the market that patients can easily become confused. They will often ask oral health educators (OHEs) what toothpastes and mouthwashes they recommend, and it is therefore important to know some background information about the most frequently used products.

TOOTHPASTE

Toothpaste comes in the form of pastes, gels or striped combinations of the two, and manufacturers compete with each other to include new ingredients in their products. There are now anti-plaque and anti-tartar agents; fluoride in

95% of pastes[1]; a range of products for sensitivity and dry mouths; whitening and anti-erosion properties, and homeopathic pastes for those seeking no chemical additives.

It is impossible to advise the OHE on what to recommend to patients – the dental professional will often be guided by what the dentist suggests and what the practice sells. If patients have always used a particular brand, they will probably be happy not to be persuaded otherwise. However, OHEs should stress the benefits of fluoride in toothpaste, particularly for children.

Children up to the age of three should use a smear of toothpaste containing 1000 ppm and adults should ensure that the paste is not swallowed in large amounts. Children over three and adults should use a pea-sized amount of toothpaste containing 1400–1500 ppm[2].

Constituents of toothpaste

Toothpaste may contain as many as 20 different ingredients, but the main ones are:

- Polishing agents – mild abrasives to remove/reduce plaque (e.g. calcium and sodium salts and gels containing silica).
- Binding agent – controls stability, consistency and dispersion of paste in the mouth (e.g. seaweed extracts, cellulose, silica).
- Foaming agent – a mild detergent that aids dispersion and psychological benefits (mouth feels clean). It is usually *sodium lauryl sulphate* (this reacts with chlorhexidine, which is why patients are advised not to use toothpaste and mouthwash at the same time).
- *Humectant* – reduces moisture loss, sweetens and keeps consistency (e.g. glycerine, sorbitol).
- Flavouring – important to consumer (often peppermint or spearmint). It can be difficult to find non-mint flavours, in which case recommend homeopathic toothpastes, which can be found in health shops.
- Therapeutic agents – fluoride. Quantities in non-prescription toothpastes are regulated to 1500 ppm maximum for adults and 1000 ppm for children under 3.

Functions of toothpaste

There are six principal functions of toothpaste (in conjunction with toothbrushing):

1. Minimises plaque and calculus build-up (plaque-removing agents). Many companies claim to have discovered agents that remove or prevent plaque

and calculus build-up. Some pastes contain chlorhexidine, which is effective but can stain. Sodium bicarbonate (baking soda) is gentler, but less effective and many patients do not like the taste.

2. Strengthening against decay (fluoride). Different forms of fluoride are present in different pastes, the most common being *sodium monofluorophosphate*. Some pastes contain sodium fluoride or stannous fluoride (the first fluoride paste produced in the 1970s contained stannous fluoride[3]).

3. Removing food debris. Many patients like the foaming action of toothpaste caused by mild detergents (usually sodium lauryl sulphate). It is important to stress that an effective method of brushing is equally important in removing food particles.

4. Freshening the mouth. Various agents are added to flavour and sweeten pastes (sugar was once used!). Now sweeteners are used: usually soluble saccharin or xylitol and flavourings as mentioned previously.

5. Desensitising (strontium chloride/potassium chloride). Statistics show that 30% of patients complain of tooth sensitivity (usually seen in those between 25 years-middle-age)[1]. Desensitising toothpastes are popular and widely used.

6. Whitening. Patients invariably want whiter teeth and may ask the OHE's advice. It should be explained that whatever the toothpaste manufacturer's claim, these toothpastes do not change the colour of teeth, but assist in removing extrinsic protein stains. If a patient is very concerned about the colour of their teeth, suggest a consultation with the dentist.

Advising on toothpastes

When advising on toothpastes at the request of a patient:

- Promote a good quality paste with fluoride.

- Be aware of different ingredients in pastes which claim to reduce plaque (patients will ask for advice on this).

- Be prepared to recommend pastes to help sensitivity (patients often ask how they work and this should be explained in simple terms).

- Be aware of homeopathic toothpastes (some patients will ask about these and they can be obtained from health shops). It is now possible to obtain homeopathic toothpaste with added fluoride. The patient must be warned that they do not always contain fluoride. If not, the patient should use a daily fluoride mouthwash to combat the loss. These pastes are often manufactured without mint or other strong flavours, which many patients find more acceptable.

ANTI-PLAQUE MOUTHWASHES

An anti-plaque mouthwash is an agent that is capable of reducing gingivitis. A claim for plaque reduction alone or having an effect on plaque will not necessarily mean it will be sufficient to reduce gum disease. It is important to look for proportional differences in claims.

Besides the treatment of gingivitis, mouthwashes can also be used as an adjunct for the treatment of periodontitis (acute and chronic), *pericoronitis*, dental caries, sensitivity and other more serious conditions of the oral mucosa. Chlorhexidine gluconate is considered the *gold standard* by which all other mouthwashes are measured.

Chlorhexidine gluconate

Chlorhexidine gluconate has a broad antimicrobial spectrum and is active on both gram-positive and gram-negative bacteria. Research has shown it to be less effective on biofilms[4].

It has been shown in long-term studies[1] to reduce plaque and gingivitis by an average of 55 and 45% respectively. Thirty per cent of a chlorhexidine gluconate mouthwash is retained in the mouth, and elevated levels are found in saliva after 24 h.

Forms of chlorhexidine gluconate

Forms of chlorhexidine gluconate include:

- Mouthwash (0.2% chlorhexidine gluconate) – rinse for 1 min every 12 h. Several mouthwashes on the market contain chlorhexidine gluconate and there is an alcohol-free chlorhexidine mouthwash; following public concern that alcohol in mouthwashes could cause cancer.
- Gel (1% chlorhexidine gluconate) – applied topically.
- Spray (0.2% chlorhexidine gluconate).
- Chewing gum.
- Toothpaste.
- Slow release chip (e.g. Periochip®) – placed in deep pockets by the dentist or hygienist.

When advising patients about the use of chlorhexidine gluconate mouthwash, they should be told to leave a gap of 60 min before toothbrushing. This is because the reaction between chlorhexidine gluconate and sodium lauryl sulphate in toothpaste reduces the effect of the mouthwash.

ANTI-PLAQUE AGENTS

Chlorhexidine gluconate usage

Chlorhexidine gluconate should be used:

- As an adjunct for periodontal therapy, for mentally or physically disabled, or medically compromised patients.
- Where plaque control is inadequate or difficult after surgery.
- In cases of recurrent ulceration.

Side effects of chlorhexidine gluconate usage

Side effects of using chlorhexidine gluconate include:

- Black/brown staining of material left on the tooth. (If it does not stain it is not working, or the patient is not using it.) Gel form should be broken up and foamed around the mouth to have an effect.
- Loss of taste.
- Increased calculus formation (long-term use, although there is a reduction in short-term use).
- Parotid swelling (rare).

Listerine® produces a phenolic, anti-plaque mouthwash with anti-inflammatory properties. This has a moderate clinical effect with reductions of 35% for both plaque and gingivitis[1]. It can be used as a *maintenance mouthwash* after periodontal treatment and is useful for patients who need an agent which will not stain to maintain their gingival improvement.

Fluoride mouthwashes

Fluoride has certain antibacterial properties and is found in varying amounts in most rinses.

Several fluoride mouthwashes have been shown to reduce caries by between 25 and 50%[1]. They can be used either once daily with a 0.05% sodium fluoride solution or once weekly rinsing with 0.2% sodium fluoride solution. In both cases, a 10 mL solution should be rinsed around the oral cavity for 1 min.

Fluoride mouthwash usage

Fluoride mouthwashes are particularly useful for:

- Prevention of caries in high risk patients
- Patients undergoing orthodontic therapy

- Preventing root caries in older people
- Patients with sensitive teeth

Hydrogen peroxide mouthwashes

Hydrogen peroxide mouthwashes (e.g. Peroxyl®) produce an oxygenated environment which hinders the function of anaerobic bacteria. They should be used for no more than 7 days at one time, and for the initial treatment of necrotising ulcerative gingivitis (NUG) and pericoronitis around partially erupted wisdom teeth.

Sodium bicarbonate

This old-fashioned remedy, now used in some toothpastes, has a neutralizing effect on acid. When dentrifices first became available early in the twentieth century, they were very expensive and people relied upon salt, bicarbonate of soda and even soot to clean their teeth. A sodium bicarbonate mouthwash can be used to quickly restore the pH of the mouth to normal after vomiting (pregnancy, bulimics).

Benzydamine hydrochloride

Benzydamine hydrochloride (0.15% concentration) comes in either mouthwash or spray form, and is often prescribed to patients following radiotherapy for pain relief and inflammation of the throat and mouth. In mouthwash form, 15 mL should be rinsed every 1.5–3 h, for no more than 7 days unless under medical supervision.

Sanguinaria

Sanguinaria is a plant alkaloid with a high affinity for plaque, although long-term studies have shown that it does not cause significant plaque or calculus reduction[1].

Cetylpyridinium chloride

Cetylpyridinium chloride is found in many mouthwashes, and claims have been made about its ability to reduce plaque and gingivitis, but long-term studies have shown it to cause a small reduction in plaque and a 24% reduction in gingivitis[1].

ANTI-PLAQUE AGENTS

SUGAR-FREE CHEWING GUM

Sugar-free chewing gum has the following benefits:

- Increases saliva flow to wash away debris
- Raises pH of plaque

SELF-ASSESSMENT

1. Define an anti-plaque agent and list the three main types.

2. What percentage of toothpastes contains fluoride?

3. List the six functions of toothpaste.

4. What percentage of chlorhexidine gluconate in mouthwashes is recommended in a daily mouthwash to treat gingivitis?

5. Which patients would you recommend use this mouthwash and how often should they rinse?

6. What possible side effects of chlorhexidine would you warn patients about?

7. What is the percentage of chlorhexidine gluconate in the gel used in the treatment of gingivitis?

8. What is the percentage of chlorhexidine gluconate in sprays recommended for some patients?

9. Why should patients not rinse with chlorhexidine gluconate immediately after using toothpaste?

10. Which mouthwash would you recommend for maintenance after ceasing the use of chlorhexidine?

11. What is the percentage of caries reduction in people who use a fluoride mouthwash?

12. What percentage and dose of fluoride mouthwash is recommended for daily and weekly use?

13. Which patients would you recommend to use a fluoride mouthwash?

14. When would you suggest a hydrogen peroxide mouthwash?

15. List the benefits of sugar-free chewing gum.

REFERENCES

1. Collins, W.J., Walsh, T., Figures, K. (1999) *A Handbook for Dental Hygienists*, 4th edn. Butterworth Heinemann, Oxford.
2. Levine, R.S., Stillman-Lowe, C.R. (2004) *The Scientific Basis of Oral Health Education*. BDJ Books, London.
3. Fejerskov, O., Kidd, E. (2004) *Dental Caries, The Disease and Its Clinical Management*. Blackwell Munksgaard, Oxford.
4. Tilling, E. (2007) *What Works and Why?* Lecture given at Gloucester Independent Hygienists' Study Day, Berkley, Gloucestershire, 16 March 2007.

ANTI-PLAQUE AGENTS

Chapter 19

Practical oral hygiene instruction

LEARNING OUTCOMES

By the end of this chapter you should be able to:

1. Motivate patients to improve plaque control.
2. Explain *disclosing*.
3. Advise patients on suitable toothbrushes.
4. Discuss the advantages and disadvantages of various toothpastes.
5. Demonstrate suitable toothbrushing techniques.
6. Give practical instruction in interdental cleaning.

INTRODUCTION

Practical oral hygiene instruction (OHI) forms a vital part of the role of an oral health educator (OHE).

In order to gain confidence in giving instruction and practical help to patients, the OHE needs to understand the theories of tooth cleaning and continually update their knowledge about both existing and new cleaning materials available.

UK law is ambiguous on whether a dental nurse can put toothbrushes and other cleaning aids in patients' mouths. A good guideline for the OHE is to have written instructions from their dental surgeon on what they are allowed to carry out. It is also courteous to ask patients if you may demonstrate toothbrushing and flossing in the mouth. If they are agreeable, avoid procedures which could cause trauma such as wire bottle brushes and wood sticks. UK law does not allow dental nurses to use instruments in patients' mouths, as this constitutes *practising dentistry*.

Good communication skills with both the dentist and the patient should enable the OHE to determine which aids can be demonstrated in the mouth.

TEACHING PLAQUE CONTROL SKILLS

Research shows[1-3] that whilst effective plaque control alone has little effect on the caries rate, it is the single most important method of preventing periodontal disease. (In the prevention of caries, other factors such as diet, fissure sealing and fluoride are also involved.)

In a practical OHI session, the OHE must be able to:

- Motivate patients to improve plaque control

- Explain and demonstrate *disclosing*

- Advise on the most suitable toothbrush for their use

- Demonstrate suitable toothbrushing techniques

- Discuss the advantages and disadvantages of various toothpastes

- Give practical instruction in interdental cleaning

Patient motivation

Communication skills are heavily involved in motivation, although the OHE will also need:

- Time to talk to the patient and find out background information

- A relaxed, unhurried approach

- Empathy with patient difficulties and problems

- Regular appointments to assess progress

- Endless patience

Disclosing

Demonstrating the use of disclosing tablets is a good way of enabling patients to identify plaque. However, it is important to remember that although disclosing tablets only stain teeth and oral structures temporarily, many adult patients will find having their mouths disclosed embarrassing. You will probably obtain a better response by showing pictures that illustrate the effects of disclosing tablets and giving the patient samples to try at home.

Suggest that the patient uses disclosing tablets:

- Regularly – perhaps once a week until plaque-removing skills improve.

- After brushing and interdental cleaning to highlight difficult areas.

PRACTICAL ORAL HYGIENE INSTRUCTION

- At a suitable time of day (e.g. not when they are about to go out).
- Apply a thin smear of petroleum jelly (e.g. Vaseline®) to lips prior to disclosing, to prevent staining.

There are various disclosing agents available, although the common active ingredient is *erythrocin* (a harmless, tasteless, red food dye). Two-tone tablets are also available and these stain *fresh* and *older* plaque different colours. These are popular with children, who often find disclosing a fun method of improving brushing.

When advising children, you must involve the parent and explain the correct use of tablets, and that it can be a messy procedure.

Toothbrushes

Advise patients on a suitable choice of toothbrush. There are so many toothbrushes on the market now that it is difficult to know which one to advise. Many dental practices sell specific brand names and the OHE will probably use brushes from the range stocked for demonstration purposes.

It is more important to ensure that patients clean their mouths effectively than to insist on a particular toothbrush or paste being used.

Remember when advising on toothbrushes:

- Suggest a good quality, medium-textured brush with nylon filaments and a small enough head to suit the patient.
- Suggest a simple design (often more effective).
- Remind the patient to change a brush when filaments show signs of wear.

Rechargeable electric toothbrushes

These toothbrushes have become increasingly popular, and the OHE should be able to demonstrate their use. This is probably best done on mouth models, but it can be helpful to let the patient feel the action of the brush on a fingernail (the demonstration brush-head can be autoclaved or cold-sterilised at the end of the session, as it is not likely to be used in the mouth).

When demonstrating the brush on mouth models, stress that particular attention should be paid to lingual, palatal and buccal surfaces of molars (the most difficult to reach) – using layman's terms. Tell the patient that if a mechanical toothbrush is being used, there is still a need for daily interdental cleaning. Modern models now have an interdental brush head, but it is only suitable for large gaps between teeth. It is also helpful around lingual margins and to reach behind upper molars.

Remind patients that heads need to be changed every 2–3 months (or before, if signs of wear are noticed).

Toothbrushing

It is now recognised that formalised toothbrushing instruction is not the best method of enabling patients to carry out effective plaque removal. It is more important to instruct patients in a method appropriate to the size and shape of their mouths and manual dexterity.

Before deciding upon the most effective brushing technique for the patient, OHEs should be able to advise on a suitable choice of toothbrush and toothpaste and suggest frequency of brushing (which may vary from patient to patient).

There are many different methods of toothbrushing. Some are designed to clean specific areas of the mouth, and some are more difficult to master than others.

The OHE should take into account the patient's:

- Needs – what is their plaque control like? Is gingivitis or periodontitis present?

- Time – will the patient spend time on a particular technique?

- Manual dexterity – not all patients can cope with certain techniques.

Frequently used techniques

Frequently used toothbrush techniques include:

1. *Bass technique/modified Bass* (Figure 19.1). The toothbrush is placed with the filaments at a 45° angle to the gingival crevice. A gentle, circular movement is designed to remove bacteria from the crevice, but requires considerable dexterity and not all patients can cope. In modified Bass, the action ends by rolling the brush down in an occlusal direction.

2. *Charter's technique* (Figure 19.2). Developed in an attempt to clean *interproximal* surfaces more efficiently, and particularly important when interdental papillae have been lost (NUG). The brush is placed at the gingival margin with filaments pointing downwards towards the occlusal surface and vibrated into the interdental spaces. Difficult to perform in lingual areas.

3. *Fones (circular) technique* (Figure 19.3). Particularly appropriate for children as it is easy and teaches them to brush the gingivae as well as teeth. The teeth are held in occlusion and large circular movements performed. The child must then be shown how to clean the lingual and occlusal surfaces

(a)

(b)

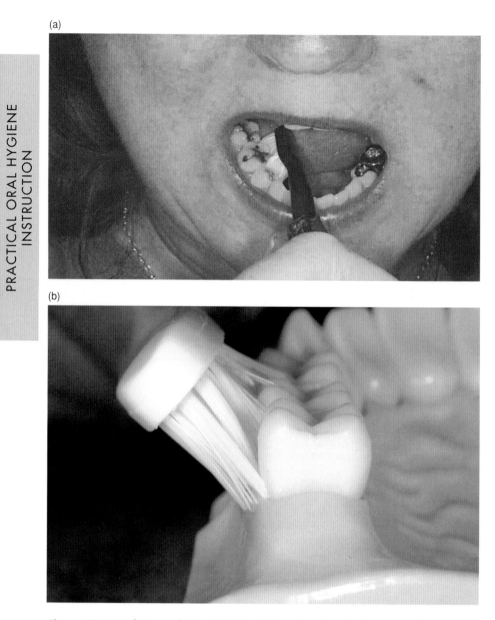

Figure 19.1 (a & b) Bass technique (© Dr Ian Bellamy. Reproduced with permission)

with a gentle scrubbing action. With a very small child, it is a good idea to make them sit on the floor, with their back to the parent, who is sitting on a chair and holding the child between his or her knees. Tilt the chin gently upwards so that a good view is obtained, then perform the technique as described.

(a)

(b)

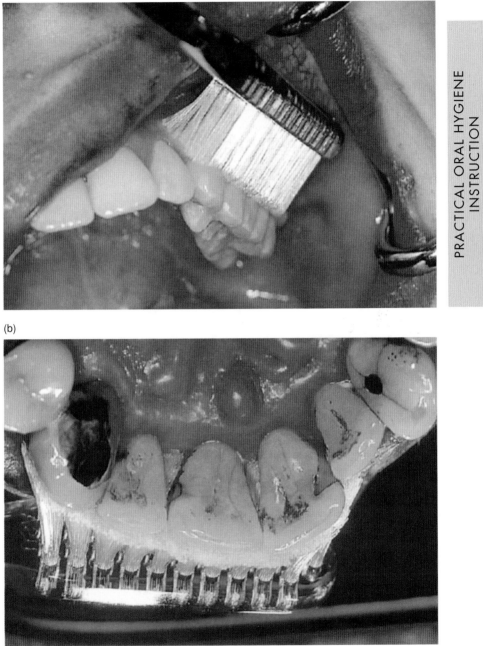

Figure 19.2 (a & b) Charter's technique (© Blackwell Publishing 2003. Reproduced with permission from Reference 4)

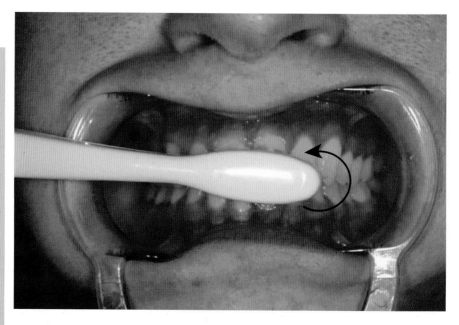

Figure 19.3 Fones (circular) technique (© Alison Chapman)

4. *Vertical technique.* Designed to prevent damage caused by horizontal scrubbing. The brush is moved up and down on buccal surfaces with the teeth in occlusion. As with Fone's technique, the disadvantage is that a different method must be used on other surfaces.

5. *Brushing with a power brush* (Figure 19.4). Work systematically around the mouth, one tooth at a time, holding the brush so that the gingival margins are gently included. Be sure to take in the lingual aspects of lower molars and buccal/distal aspects of upper molars. Complete the brushing by gently sunning the brush along the occlusal surface.

Whichever technique is used, it is a good idea to demonstrate on a model, then give the patient a brush and ask for a repeat demonstration on the model and in the mouth. If the patient is removing plaque effectively, do not try to change the toothbrushing technique. It may be a combination of all of the above methods but if it is effective – this does not matter.

Interdental cleaning methods

Most patients are well aware of the importance of toothbrushing, but many are still not cleaning interdental areas regularly, and do not realise that this is vital in preventing periodontal disease.

(a)

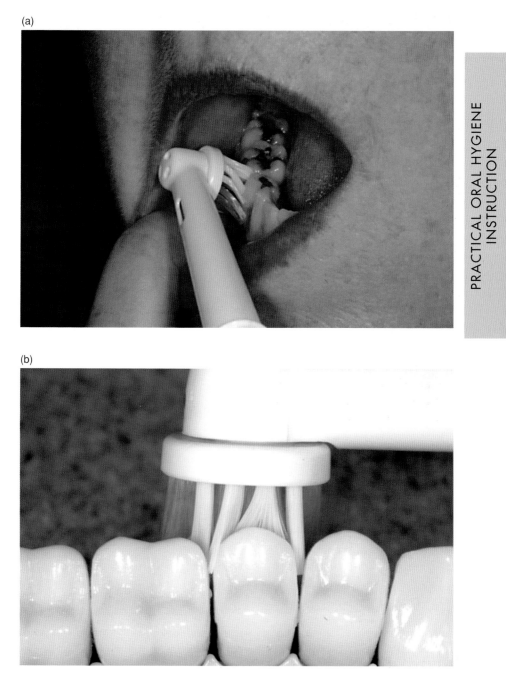

(b)

Figure 19.4 (a & b) Power brush technique (© Dr Ian Bellamy. Reproduced with permission)

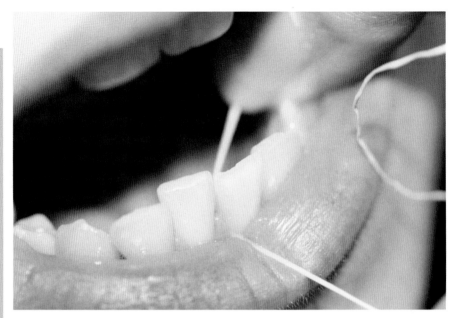

Figure 19.5 Interdental plaque removal (using floss) (© Carole Hollins. Reproduced with permission from Reference 5)

OHEs must be able to advise on the different methods available and suggest the most suitable for each patient, including floss and tape, interdental and *bottle* brushes, wood sticks and water irrigation units.

Floss and tape

If used effectively, floss and tape are probably the most efficient methods of interdental plaque removal (Figure 19.5).

The OHE should be aware of the different types of floss, such as waxed and unwaxed, and patients should be encouraged to try different types of floss and tape, to see which they prefer.

Those who dislike the idea of floss may be persuaded to try tape, which is flat rather than rounded and slides more easily into tight contact areas. Floss picks are helpful for people who only have the use of one hand or limited manual dexterity.

Demonstrate flossing on a model and show pictures or diagrams of the correct technique, then encourage the patient to demonstrate their skill.

Interdental and bottle brushes

Patients who do not like floss or tape will often cope better with brushes (Figure 19.6). There are many on the market (with long or short handles), and they

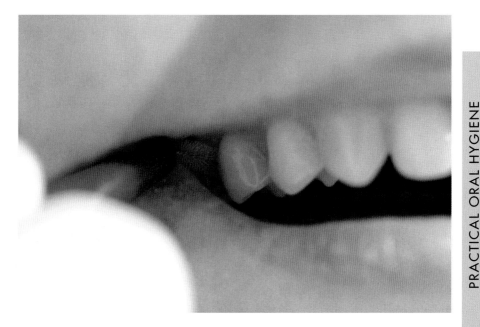

Figure 19.6 Bottle brush usage (© Carole Hollins. Reproduced with permission from Reference 5)

are particularly effective on large interdental spaces where patients should be encouraged to use the largest brush head possible.

Great care should be taken when demonstrating brushes with central wire shanks, as these can traumatise gingivae. (If possible, show the patient a picture of someone using the brush and demonstrate on models.) Several makes of interdental brushes now have a plastic covering on the central metal spine to prevent scratching of titanium implants.

Wood sticks

Wood sticks are also a popular method of interdental cleaning, particularly with older patients, who will often not use floss. They are less efficient than floss, but quicker to use, and so appropriate for less motivated patients. Once again, patients can be shown pictures of their use or the OHE can demonstrate on a model.

Water irrigation units

Patients see these units advertised and often ask about them. They are expensive and inefficient at removing plaque, so are not to be recommended.

SELF-ASSESSMENT EXERCISES

Exercise 1

1. Disclose your own mouth, after eating a meal (of fairly sticky foods) and before brushing your teeth.
2. Gently remove some plaque, using floss or tape.
3. Look at the plaque and try to remember what it consists of.
4. Look at a picture of plaque.
5. Brush and floss your teeth in front of a mirror, until no trace of plaque remains.
6. Disclose your mouth again, to see if you have succeeded in your own oral health procedures – you may be surprised at how difficult it is to remove plaque effectively.

Exercise 2

Now you can move on and test your skills on someone else.

1. Find an obliging friend or relative who will help you to check your learning.
2. Put® on Vaseline on their lips (to minimise staining), then help the patient disclose the plaque.
3. Explain what *plaque* is to your patient in simple terms that a non-dental person would understand
4. Ask if your explanation was easy to understand.
5. Take note of patient comments (i.e. *patient evaluation*).

Exercise 3

1. Find a dentally trained colleague.
2. Using your dental knowledge and technical jargon, explain the development of plaque from the salivary pellicle stage to mature plaque.
3. Ask for feedback and constructive criticism on your performance.
4. Do not be offended if you were not perfect – read this chapter again and have another try.

REFERENCES

1. Fejerskov, O., Kidd, E. (2004) *Dental Caries, The Disease and Its Clinical Management*. Blackwell Munksgaard, Oxford.
2. Lindhe, J., Karring, T., Lang, N. (2003) *Clinical Periodontology and Implant Dentistry*, 4th edn. Blackwell Munksgaard, Oxford.
3. Levine, R.S., Stillman, C.R. (2004) *The Scientific Basis of Oral Health Education*, British Dental Journal. BDJ Books, London.
4. Echeverría, J.J., Sanz, M. (2003) *Mechanical Supragingival Plaque Control*. In Lindhe, J., Karring, T. Lang, N.P. (Eds): *Clinical Periodontology and Implant Dentistry*, 4th edn, pp. 449–463. Blackwell Munksgaard, Oxford.
5. Hollins, C. (2008) *Basic Guide to Dental Procedures*. Wiley Blackwell, Oxford.

SECTION 5

ORAL HEALTH TARGET GROUPS AND CASE STUDIES

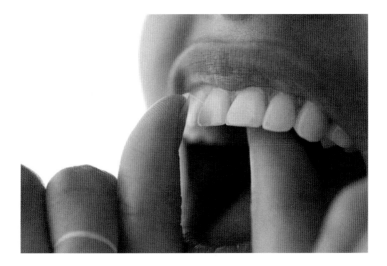

This section mainly concerns delivering oral health education to *target groups* – specific patient types at the receiving end of oral health education. It advises on the particular problems which may be encountered when dealing with patients who need specialized care and attention from dental professionals for a number of reasons.

The section concludes with a chapter particularly aimed at nurses taking the NEBDN exam, detailing points to remember when planning and carrying out case studies and an exhibition (based on patients from target groups).

Chapter 20

Pregnant and nursing mothers

LEARNING OUTCOMES

By the end of this chapter you should be able to:

1. Confidently discuss dental issues and conditions related to pregnancy and baby care with the patient (including the mother's diet and care of an infant's teeth).

2. List the signs and symptoms of *pregnancy gingivitis*

3. Explain the risks to mother and baby of smoking during pregnancy, the nursing period and beyond.

INTRODUCTION

Pregnant women and nursing mothers (i.e. mothers of babies of up to 1 year old) are an important target group. Good dental advice and care during and following pregnancy are important to avoid permanent gingival damage. An increased risk of caries and tooth erosion can result from morning sickness.

THE ROLE OF THE OHE

The OHE's role is to explain changes that pregnant/nursing mothers may have noticed in the health of their mouths, and to give advice and reassurance.

Pregnant women are generally very receptive to information and keen to do the best they can for their health and that of the coming baby. During routine antenatal care, they are encouraged to seek dental advice, and many, who are not regular dental attenders, will attend during pregnancy for the sake of the coming child. They are encouraged further in the UK as NHS practices offer free NHS treatment to pregnant women and children. However, it is often difficult to register with an NHS practice and many pregnant patients therefore opt to stay with their private practice.

The OHE may be surprised to find that some women (usually those in areas of social deprivation who have only visited the dentist as a result of antenatal advice) are still unaware of the need for good oral hygiene and dental care during pregnancy. They will perhaps have heard *old wives' tales* from friends and relatives such as 'lose a tooth for every child' and 'the developing baby takes calcium from the mother's teeth'. The role of the OHE is to dispel these myths and to help patients develop an effective oral health routine, which they can continue as their family grows up.

An increased intake of 'healthier' foods by pregnant women may inadvertently increase the amount of acidic drinks and foods during pregnancy, such as fruit, fruit juices and dressed salads. In order to protect the enamel of teeth from an increased risk of toothbrush abrasion and erosion, it is important to stress that toothbrushing should not be carried out immediately after eating or an episode of vomiting. The mouth should be rinsed with water only and brushing with toothpaste carried out at least 30 min after eating.

SUSCEPTIBILITY TO ORAL DISEASES AND CONDITIONS

Patients' susceptibility to the following oral diseases and conditions can increase during pregnancy.

Caries

Susceptibility to caries can increase during pregnancy, due to:

- Frequent snacking (larger appetite, known as 'eating for two').
- Cravings (often for sweet foods).
- Nausea when toothbrushing and/or a dislike of the taste of a particular toothpaste can lead to an actual reduction in frequency of toothbrushing.

As an OHE, it is important not to give out-of-date or conflicting advice. Check what dietary information other members of the health care team (e.g. midwives) are giving to a pregnant woman. Be aware of local and national initiatives such as *Healthy Start* – a UK government programme which aims to achieve better outcomes for children, parents and communities in England[1].

Gingival problems

An increased risk of gingival problems in pregnant patients is due to:

- Nausea (preventing effective oral hygiene, usually in the early weeks but may continue throughout pregnancy).
- Hormonal changes (causing an exaggerated response to plaque toxins).

Pregnancy gingivitis

Some patients may develop this worrying and uncomfortable condition that usually resolves itself once the baby is born. If untreated, it can lead to permanent damage to gums and supporting tissues. Pregnancy gingivitis is more likely to occur in women who have poor oral hygiene and/or gingival problems before pregnancy, but it can also affect women with excellent oral hygiene and hitherto healthy gums. There is an exaggerated response to dental plaque due to increased hormone activity.

Symptoms of pregnancy gingivitis

The patient may complain of:

- Bleeding on brushing – sometimes profuse and where none has occurred before.
- Spontaneous bleeding – blood on the pillow or when eating crisp foods (e.g. apple).
- Occasional irritation or 'itchiness' of the gums.
- Halitosis.

Signs of pregnancy gingivitis

The dental professional should look for:

- Increased tendency for gums to bleed on gentle probing.
- Gingivae – blue-red, shiny, swollen and smooth (due to increased vascular activity).
- *Epulis* formation (or *pregnancy tumour*) in severe cases, though rare.

An *epulis* (Figure 20.1) is a localised area of swollen interdental papilla which may or may not contain pus. It can be found anywhere in the mouth, but is most commonly seen in the anterior regions. There may be more than

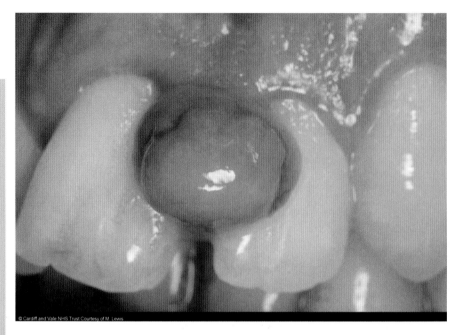

Figure 20.1 Pregnancy epulis (© Professor M.A.O. Lewis, Cardiff University. Reproduced with permission)

one present and it is important to reassure the patient that there is no likelihood of malignancy. The OHE should ensure that the dentist has seen the epulis and be able to tell the patient that it will almost certainly disappear after birth. Very occasionally, an epulis persists and surgical removal is necessary at a later date.

Even with improved oral hygiene, pregnancy gingivitis sometimes persists until breastfeeding has finished and hormone levels have returned to normal. This becomes more significant if there is a progression to periodontal disease.

Periodontal infection

Research[2] shows that untreated periodontal infection (i.e. anaerobic bacterial infection in pockets) during pregnancy can result in:

- Pre-term labour
- Premature birth
- Low birth weight

It is thought that these conditions occur because the body can only deal with so many problems at a time, and in a pregnant woman the growth of the baby can be impaired if the immune system is also dealing with periodontal infection.

Smoking and pregnancy

Smoking during pregnancy is also associated with gingival problems, because it compromises the oxygen carrying capacity of haemoglobin (carbon monoxide from cigarette smoke replaces and diminishes oxygen). Smoking also contributes to stickier plaque formation and dries the mouth[3].

Smoking during pregnancy can lead to:

- Miscarriage
- Stillbirth
- Premature membrane rupture and delivery
- *Placenta previa*
- Foetal growth restriction

Smoking in the postnatal period

Smoking during the postnatal period can lead to:

- Sudden infant death syndrome (SIDS).
- Increase in the mother's blood pressure.
- Mental retardation and behavioural, psychiatric and cognitive problems.

Smoking by parents of small children

Passive intake of smoke by children can lead to the following conditions:

- Respiratory illness
- Asthma
- *Otitis media* (middle ear infection)

SUMMARY OF ADVICE FOR PREGNANT WOMEN

The OHE should stress the following points to pregnant patients:

- Try to make time for oral care at a time of day when sickness is not present (sometimes a smaller-headed brush will help to avoid nausea when brushing).
- Use a fluoride toothpaste (there is no appreciable benefit to the developing baby in taking fluoride supplements, but fluoride paste will help prevent decay for the mother).

- Choose a softer toothbrush if gums are sore and bleeding, and use a gentle scrub or the *Bass technique*.

- Interdental care is even more important than usual (if bleeding is present, chlorhexidine mouthwash/gel may be used with interdental aids). Explain that this is not dangerous to the baby (but should be used sparingly and for as short a time as possible to avoid staining and maternal anxiety). Although stains can be removed, many pregnant women are wary of ingesting chemicals in the gestation period.

- Keep up regular dental checks and hygienist visits.

- Fluoride mouthwash may help combat the effects of nausea and frequent snacking.

- Stop smoking – many pregnant women will have stopped by themselves, but there are still some who cannot. In the UK, suggest that the patient accesses NHS smoking cessation support. Emphasise that once the baby is born, a smoke-free environment should be provided whenever possible.

Remember! The primary causes of pregnancy gingivitis and epulis formation are the enzymes and toxins of mature plaque. Hormonal change is a secondary factor. Also, remember that fathers, possibly grandparents and sometimes childminders, also share responsibility for children's oral care.

SELF-ASSESSMENT

1. Why do pregnant/nursing women make a particularly good target group for oral health education?

2. What *myths* may the OHE need to dispel?

3. List three reasons why susceptibility to caries may increase during pregnancy, and what advice would you offer to combat this?

4. Give two reasons why gingival problems are more likely to occur during pregnancy.

5. List the signs and symptoms of pregnancy gingivitis.

6. What is a *pregnancy epulis* and what is its primary cause?

7. What does recent research show concerning periodontal infection in pregnancy?

8. What reasons would you give a pregnant mother for stopping smoking?

REFERENCES

1. Healthy start. Available at www.healthystart.nhs.
2. Gallie, A. (2006) Periodontal and systemic disease – what is the link? In Action in Practice, *Wrigley Oral Healthcare in Action*, Vol. 8, No. 1.
3. Haiek, P. (2006) *Smoking Cessation Training and Research Programme (Maudsley Clinic Model)*. Park Crescent Conference Centre, London, 3–5 July 2006.

PREGNANT AND NURSING
MOTHERS

Chapter 21
Parents of pre-11-year-olds

LEARNING OUTCOMES

By the end of this chapter you should be able to:

1. Discuss eruption dates and the ongoing care of deciduous and permanent teeth with parents.
2. Give advice to parents on the appropriate use of fluoride.
3. Advise on safe snacks and drinks for children.
4. Advise parents on the importance of regular dental visits.

INTRODUCTION

Parents will often ask for help on care of their children's teeth, and parents of pre-11-year-old children are an important target group for the oral health educator (OHE).

ADVICE TO PARENTS OF 0–2-YEAR-OLDS

Parents of 0–2-year-olds are often bombarded with advice from health professionals, friends and family. However, much of this advice concerns the general well-being of the infant and parents usually welcome specific information on the following topics.

Eruption dates (see Chapter 1)

Effective cleaning of newly erupted teeth/suitable brushes

Parents should be advised to clean gently around erupting teeth with a smear of toothpaste (containing 1000 ppm fluoride) on a small piece of gauze or cotton-wool bud. Alternatively, a soft child's brush may be used from the start (if the baby is cooperative). The application of fluoride paste as soon as the teeth *erupt* is important.

Fluoride toothpaste

No more than a smear of toothpaste (containing 1000 ppm of fluoride) should be used. They should be encouraged to spit out surplus paste, rinse with a little water on the brush and avoid rinsing from a cup. It is now recognised that brushing with a fluoride paste, particularly at night, when the fluoride remains in the mouth, aids remineralisation, and is the most effective method of preventing caries in children.

Fluoride supplements

It is the responsibility of the dentist to advise on this and the OHE must follow that advice. Supplements are rarely advised now unless the patient has a high risk of caries.

Comforters

Comforters dipped in sweet substances should be avoided, and a baby should not be left alone with liquid in a bottle. This practice (apart from being unsafe) results in the constant bathing of tooth enamel in sugars and can lead to severe, rapid destruction. Research shows[1] that the prolonged use of a bottle and certain infant drinking cups can result in *bottle caries*. Only milk or water should be given in a bottle.

Breast-milk substitutes

Formula breast-milk substitutes should be discussed with health visitors, and if possible the OHE should obtain information from these professionals. Note that soya milk and rice milk (sometimes recommended for allergy reasons) are high in sugar. Cartons with no added sugar can be bought for older children but they are not suitable for babies. Low fat milk is not suitable for *under twos* (fat is an important source of calories and important vitamins and minerals required at this age). Formula milk should be given alongside solid foods until at least 1 year old. Cow's milk, for drinking, should only be given after the baby is 1 year old.

Weaning and diet

The importance of reading food labels should be explained, even on specially formulated baby foods and drinks. Suggest sugar-free foods such as bread-sticks, wholemeal toast, raw carrots, celery (to chew on) and plain yoghurt with mashed banana as a snack.

Small children (like much of the population) tend to 'graze' continually, eating up to six times a day, rather than three meals as was the trend in previous generations. Sugar-free *grazing foods* should be recommended.

Gently and diplomatically suggest appropriate dietary advice to well-meaning grandparents, partners and friends. Sweet treats should be avoided where possible and only given at pre-agreed times such as immediately after a meal/once a week. Suggest investigating snacks given at nursery and playschool before the child joins.

Drinking cups

Research[2] shows concern among dental professionals about the trend to wean children from bottles on to feeder cups (especially non-spill models, sometimes referred to as 'bottles in disguise'). Parents favour feeder cups because they do not leak when dropped, but they still require a sucking action rather than normal drinking and therefore encourage constant sipping on demand – which can be detrimental to erupting teeth.

There is also concern about the effect feeder cups have on the developing muscles of the face and mouth. Parents should be strongly encouraged to wean their children on to a normal child's cup without a lid. Aim to discontinue use of a bottle after the first 12 months. Cups with lids and valves to prevent spillage also encourage continual sipping and can result in caries.

OHEs should recommend weaning babies on to a slanting *Doidy cup*[2], which is easy to use and has no lid[2], then move onto a normal cup.

Refusal of child to cooperate

Some children will refuse to cooperate with toothbrushing. Parents may mention that a hitherto cooperative baby takes delight in clamping their mouth shut at the approach of the toothbrush, once the age of two has been reached. Explain that this is a normal stage of development and usually temporary.

The best approach is to ignore the rebellion and try to create diversions, such as new toothbrushes and brushing charts/competitions/games/rewards for older siblings. If there are no older children, parents can try brushing their own teeth (and making it look like fun!) in front of the little rebel. Forcing the issue is rarely effective.

ADVICE TO PARENTS OF CHILDREN AGED 2–5 YEARS

The ideal time to begin dental visits is when the toddler's primary dentition is complete (at around 2–3 years). However, many infants are eager to show their teeth to the dentist at a much younger age and this should be encouraged.

Children between 2 and 5 years are still very dependent on parents for dental care and the OHE should be able to discuss with parents:

- Eruption dates.

- Size/type of toothbrush.

- Fluoride toothpaste (amount and strength).

- Fluoride supplements (if appropriate).

- Toothbrushing. *Fones circular technique* is very effective, but the parent must also be shown how to brush the lingual/palatal/occlusal surfaces. Sometimes it is easier to sit with a child between the knees, its back towards you, tilting the head gently upwards. A child should not be allowed to run around or be left unattended with a toothbrush in its mouth.

- Diet/drinks – it is very important to establish good habits at this age, re-membering that this age group is now mixing with peers and visiting other people's homes, where parents may not be responsible for meal planning and snacks. Providing that a varied diet is being eaten, semi-skimmed milk can be drunk from 2 years old. (Fully skimmed milk is not suitable until a child is 5 years old because it does not contain enough calories or vitamins.) Reiterate the importance of reading food labels and suggest that parents may be able to get together with friends in order to agree 'ground-rules' when giving food to each other's children. Milk or water should be advised in between meals.

- Explain that the first permanent molars (sixes) will erupt at the age of around 6–7 years, and the importance of cleaning. Patients are often unaware of these teeth erupting and think that no second teeth appear until a deciduous tooth has been lost.

ADVICE TO PARENTS OF CHILDREN AGED 6–11 YEARS

These children are becoming more independent and like to brush their own teeth. It is generally thought that parents should supervise and help with cleaning until the age of at least 7 years[3]. Many parents, however, will think it advisable to supervise all children still of primary school age.

It is a good idea to involve both parents and children at this stage. Primary school children are particularly receptive to learning, and it is easy to capture their attention and involve them in selecting toothbrushes and thinking about their diet. A good range of resources and visual aids is essential (e.g. models showing the permanent teeth erupting).

Eruption dates

Information on eruption dates is particularly important now as they begin losing deciduous teeth and permanent teeth are erupting. Also, provide information on what action should be taken if a child knocks a tooth out[4].

Suitable brushes, techniques and toothpaste

Rechargeable electric toothbrushes are particularly effective in encouraging reluctant brushers, but still require supervision. The technique is less important than effective plaque removal. Not everyone likes (or can afford) these brushes, and you should explain that an ordinary brush can be used with equal effect.

Fluoride mouthwash (if appropriate)

Fluoride mouthwashes are only suitable when the child is able to spit out, and many are not recommended for use by children under 6 years.

Diet and the significance of frequency of sugar intake

This age group is capable of understanding that sugar consumption causes tooth decay. They are receptive to alternative snacks and will enjoy taking part in games and competitions which demonstrate how much hidden sugar is consumed. The UK National Curriculum encompasses education on health matters and many teachers will welcome a health professional who is prepared to present an exhibition on safer snacks for teeth.

PARENTS OF PRE-11-YEAR-OLDS

Drinks

Drinks become an increasingly important topic in this age group as the child will be capable of obtaining their own. *Erosion* should be explained, and the importance of avoiding, where possible, frequent sipping of acidic beverages such as fresh juice, squash and carbonated drinks. Consumption of these drinks should be limited to mealtimes and ideally drunk quickly without swishing around the mouth. Drinking through a straw is recommended where practical and serving the drink chilled. (Cold drinks have a higher pH than warm drinks.)

Games

Suggest games (e.g. play foods) to encourage children to read food labels. Have leaflets and lists of hidden sugar names available. Reinforce advice for parents to read food labels.

Schools

Build links with local schools. Find out about pupil needs and abilities, and suggest checking out national policy on diet and healthy choices. Ensure sweets are not used as a reward mechanism. A visit to the school on a parents' evening would provide an opportunity for parents to receive more information. Suggest an article about oral health education in the school newsletter. Mention the promotion of mouth guards for sport. Try to link in with other health professionals, with reference to discouraging smoking by highlighting the risks to oral health. Set up an exhibition or display.

Prevention of gum disease

Parents are often focussed on preventing caries and forget about gingival health. A surprising number of children in this age group present with gingivitis and this becomes even more of a problem if an orthodontic appliance later becomes necessary. Children of this age will enjoy using disclosing tablets (but remember that it can be messy and written permission for this should be obtained from parents). Check school policy on this type of intervention especially if disclosing tablets are to be taken home.

Sugar-free medicines

Advise parents to request sugar-free medicines from doctors and pharmacies whenever possible.

'One hour before bed' rule

Encourage a 'one hour before bed' rule (i.e. no snacks or drinks 1 h before bed). Toothpaste should be the last thing on the teeth before sleep. Only water should be provided if children require drinks through the night.

SELF-ASSESSMENT

1. Write three paragraphs from memory, summarising the advice you would give to parents of children aged 0–2 years, 2–5 years and 6–11 years. Include brief advice on eruption dates, diet, toothbrushing, fluoride and dental visits.

REFERENCES

1. Bowen, W.H., Lawrence, R.A. (2005) Comparison of the cariogenicity of cola, honey, cow milk, human milk, and sucrose, *Paediatrics*, 116(Supp. 4), 921–926.
2. National Childbirth Trust. Available at www.nctms.co.uk.
3. Levine, R.S., Stillman, C.R. (2004) *The Scientific Basis of Oral Health Education*, British Dental Journal. BDJ Books, London.
4. Blinkhorn, A.S., Mackie, I. (2007) *Prevent a Child Losing a Smile*. Colgate-Palmolive Company, Guildford.

PARENTS OF PRE-11-YEAR-OLDS

Chapter 22

Adolescents and orthodontic patients

LEARNING OUTCOMES

By the end of this chapter you should be able to:

1. Use knowledge to motivate adolescent patients towards improved oral health (including specific advice during orthodontic treatment).

2. Advise on healthy snacks and drinks.

3. Explain which *fluoride-containing* products should be used.

4. Demonstrate the care of orthodontic appliances.

5. Briefly explain and differentiate between *Angle's classes*.

ADOLESCENTS

Between 11 and 19 years, young people begin to assume control of and take responsibility for their lives. Changing to secondary education at around 11 years of age is regarded as a milestone in the UK, and children begin to challenge parental control and involvement in their general well-being.

By the mid-teenage years, adolescents have a full adult dentition (except for wisdom teeth), and may present with the same problems as adults (i.e. gingivitis and caries as well as erosion).

Young people in this target group will have opinions on what and when they eat. Peer pressure is strong, and in order to be part of the crowd snacking or *grazing* tends to be preferred. Media influence can play a large part in determining what the latest trend will be. Adolescents also go through growth spurts during these years and are frequently hungry between meals.

Treating adolescents

When dealing with this age group the OHE should remember the following points:

- It is best to tackle one problem at a time (e.g. gingivitis). Dealing with too many problems at once is impractical for the professional and too much for the patient to cope with.

- Target the young person rather than the parent (be tactful and remember that the parents may wish to be involved or kept informed). However, in the UK, it is the choice of the young person as to whether or not the parent is in the surgery with them following a House of Lords court ruling in 1985[1].

- Never patronise or 'talk down' to teenagers. Treat them as adults and they will usually respond appropriately.

- Try to find acceptable methods of communication/motivation – it may be more difficult to motivate boys, particularly in their early teens. Girls of this age are already concerned about their appearance, which can be a powerful motivational tool. Boys may respond to dental advice if it can be related to TV or sports heroes.

- Remember that peer groups have an important part to play at this age – talking to adolescents in school or uniformed groups often works well and teachers/leaders may welcome dental talks as health care is included in the UK National Curriculum. Advice can be associated with 'badge work' in groups like scouts and guides.

- *Intra-oral* mouth piercing should be discouraged. Tongue bars and balls are known to damage both upper and lower central incisors. If already in situ then oral health instruction will be required.

- Be aware of bulimia and anorexia – look for signs (e.g. weight obsession and tooth erosion). Erosion in this situation is commonly seen on palatal and lingual surfaces and the dentist may be the first health professional to identify a possible 'eating disorder'. Careful and sensitive management is required.

Advice for adolescents

Advice for adolescents should include the following topics[2].

Effective cleaning

Advice on effective cleaning should include:

- Toothbrushing – teenagers can usually cope with the *Bass technique*, but be flexible and do not insist on a particular technique if the patient is cleaning effectively.

- Toothbrushes – many teenagers use rechargeable electric brushes. Be prepared to demonstrate the use of these and advise on ordinary toothbrushes (size, texture, and frequency of renewal).

- Toothpaste (a fluoride paste is important) – check whether too much is being used. Many adolescents are avid watchers of TV adverts, where large amounts of toothpaste being squeezed onto brushes is often shown and copied.

- Interdental cleaning – now is a good time to establish a routine and most people over 11 years can be taught to use floss. Explain why interdental cleaning is vital (using pictures or commercial leaflets). Bottle brushes, if carefully used, can be an acceptable alternative, particularly when an orthodontic appliance is in place.

Dietary advice

Advice on diet should include:

- The importance of a balanced diet – low in extrinsic sugars and healthy snacks and drinks.

- Chewing a sugar-free gum between meals – particularly after school lunch or break-time snacks when brushing is not practical (school policy on gum and wearing of orthodontic appliances must be taken into consideration).

- Fashionable snacks. Adolescents should be made aware of the potential harm to the oral cavity and general health of the following fashionable foods:

  - Chocolate, biscuits and cakes.

  - Cereal bars – often high in sugar, though designed to look filling and healthy.

  - Crisps and savoury snacks – some are high in sugar and labels should be studied.

  - Fizzy drinks (e.g. cola). It is the *done thing* to sip these, thus maintaining contact with teeth over long periods.

  - Sports drinks – also have high sugar content.

  - Diet drinks – contain preservatives such as citric and phosphoric acid in place of sugar. These are one of the main causes of the dramatic increase in tooth erosion seen by dentists in recent years (seen on the labial and incisal aspects of upper central incisors).

Fluoride

Systemic fluoride is likely to have less effect in adolescents than in smaller children, but topical fluorides are still important and include:

- Toothpaste – be prepared to explain how it works.
- Mouthwashes – important if there is a high decay rate or an orthodontic appliance is being worn.

Regular dental/orthodontic checkups

Remember that until now most youngsters have attended the dentist regularly in family groups. When they leave home for university or take responsibility for their own lives, regular dental attendance may lapse. Therefore, stress the importance of:

- Regular check-ups (even if seeing orthodontist regularly)
- Hygienist visits if referred by dentist

Anti-smoking advice

An early teen is also a good time to give anti-smoking information (as many adolescents take up the habit).

Oral piercing advice

Tongue and other oral piercings have become fashionable in recent years. The OHE should advise on oral hygiene procedures if a patient has piercings or is considering them and should provide the following advice[3]:

- Find a reputable practitioner prior to piercing (consult the European Professional Piercers' Association).
- Brush tongue, studs and barbells twice daily with a soft toothbrush.
- Remove studs monthly, clean thoroughly and check regularly to make sure intact.
- Do not use ordinary jewellery cleaners (irritant properties).
- Take care when eating and do not fiddle or play with studs.
- If infection, swallowing or breathing difficulties occur, seek urgent medical help.
- Visit dentist if a tooth is chipped or damaged by a stud.

ADOLESCENTS AND ORTHODONTIC PATIENTS

Sports guards

Promote sports guards, which can be made in 'team colours' or designs. Also promote the use of water rather than sports drinks unless specific training needs have to be met.

THE ORTHODONTIC PATIENT

Orthodontics describes the treatment of malalignment conditions of the teeth.

The need for treatment is based on preventive, cosmetic and functional considerations.

Although, as an OHE, you will not be expected to understand why orthodontic treatment is carried out and how it works, background information is useful.

Many adolescents have orthodontic appliances (Figure 22.1). Be prepared to give advice on care and cleaning of appliances and efficient mouth cleaning whilst the appliance is in place – including interdental cleaning and the use of fluoride mouthwash.

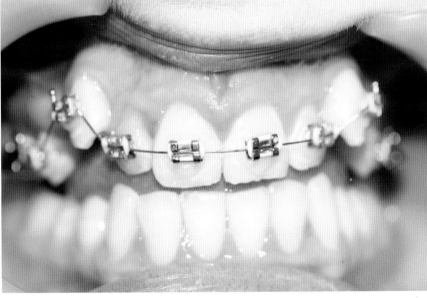

Figure 22.1 Mouth with orthodontic fixed appliances (© Carole Hollins. Reproduced with permission from Reference 4)

Treatment of the orthodontic patient

The orthodontist will take the following points into consideration when determining treatment:

- Skeletal pattern.

- Occlusion (i.e. how the upper and lower teeth meet). When assessing this, the true positions of the maxilla and mandible are taken into account. Measurements are taken to determine whether it is the jaws or the teeth in the alveolus that are misplaced. A lateral skull radiograph is taken to assist diagnosis. This shows the bones of the skull from the side and the use of a filter allows the shadow of the soft tissues to be seen.

- Teeth. Two patterns (molar and incisal relationships) are considered. The position of the teeth is classified by *Angle's classes*, which define the terms *overbite* and *overjet*:

  - Overbite: how the lower incisors bite into the uppers

  - Overjet: the horizontal relationship (how the teeth stick out)

Angle's classifications

Angle's classification is used to describe the relationship of the molars in occlusion[5]. Dental nurse students using orthodontic patients as case studies may wish to go into this in more detail[5].

Class I

Normal relationship where lower 6 cusp tip bites half a cusp width in front of upper 6. The overjet and overbite are 2–4 mm.

Class II

The lower 6 is less than half a cusp tip width in front of upper 6. Upper centrals are in front of lowers. This class has two divisions:

- Division 1 (known as Class II, div 1). Upper teeth are much further forward than lowers, usually because of overcrowding. This tends to accentuate the upper teeth, the upper anteriors being *proclined* (protruding).

- Division 2 (known as Class II, div 2). Overcrowding causes upper incisors to *retrocline* (lean back) and sometimes the lowers also. Typically, the laterals overlap centrals and cause problems as there is nothing to restrain the lower anteriors that over-erupt and bite into the palate, while upper incisors bite into the labial gingivae. Lower anteriors can give an 'organ pipe' appearance.

Class III

Lower teeth are in front of the uppers, with the lower 6 more than half a cusp tip width forward. The bite is either edge to edge, or a reverse overbite. This can be due to oversized lower teeth, stunted maxillary growth, or overgrowth of the mandible.

Advice for the orthodontic patient

Advice should be given for either removable or fixed appliances, and special consideration should be given to each.

Removable appliances

Removable appliances should be worn at all times – unless advised otherwise by an orthodontist. When not being used they should be kept in water in a special orthodontic box.

Advise cleaning twice daily at the same time as normal toothbrushing. Hold the appliance in the palm of the hand over a basin of water and brush with soapy water using a soft toothbrush or a soft nailbrush. Take care to remove all food debris and plaque from around the wires/springs. Suggest weekly disclosing before removing the appliance to highlight problem areas. Rinse carefully and replace. The appliance can also be removed and rinsed after eating.

Patients should also avoid very hard and sticky foods (e.g. toffees, chewing gum). Fizzy drinks and fruit juices should only be drunk at mealtimes.

Broken or lost appliances should be reported to the orthodontist as soon as possible – preferably the same day. An excellent standard of toothbrushing should be maintained and stress the importance of gingival health whilst the appliance is being worn. Daily interdental cleaning is also vital.

Fixed appliances

Adolescents usually adapt to wearing these surprisingly well and quickly, but they need careful advice on keeping the appliance and natural teeth clean to avoid gum problems – advise a special orthodontic brush or a small headed, medium/soft texture brush.

Promote the use of fluoride toothpaste. Some patients may do well with an rechargeable electric brush, particularly if using one already. Great care must be taken around brackets, bands and wires. An interdental brush can also be useful. Help may be required with bottle brushes and if there is suitable space, guidance on inserting them carefully.

The use of a fluoride mouthwash can help to avoid demineralisation around brackets and should be carried out at a different time to brushing.

As for diet, stress the usual dietary advice with reference to snacking, avoiding sugars wherever possible and difficult-to-eat foodstuffs (e.g. toffees, chewing gum). For drinks, the same advice applies as to *adolescents*, and also encourage the use of straws.

Patients should attend orthodontic/dental check-ups and report discomfort promptly. Patients may be given dental wax to use on any wires which may traumatise the buccal mucosa. It is important that, should a bracket become loose, advice is sought from the orthodontist.

Retainers should be fitted after active treatment to prevent relapse (teeth moving back in original position). These should be worn as recommended by the orthodontist. Some patients will have fixed retainers usually behind the anterior teeth, which will need careful cleaning as they can become food traps and susceptible to calculus build-up.

SELF-ASSESSMENT

1. An adolescent presents with erosion caused by carbonated drinks. What methods would you use to influence his/her lifestyle in addressing this problem?

2. Discuss the advice you would give to an adolescent who has just been fitted with a fixed orthodontic appliance. How would you vary your advice if the appliance fitted were removable?

REFERENCES

1. Wheeler, R. (April 2006) Gillick or fraser? A plea for consistency over competence in children, *British Medical Journal*, 332(7545), 807.
2. Levine, R.S., Stillman, C.R. (2004) *The Scientific Basis of Oral Health Education*, British Dental Journal. BDJ Books, London.
3. Wrigley, Tongue Piercing, Advice on Mouth Piercing, *Oral Healthcare in Action*, Handout 21. Available at www.betteroralhealth.info.
4. Hollins, C. (2008) *Basic Guide to Dental Procedures*, Wiley Blackwell, Oxford.
5. Ireland, R. (2004) *Advanced Dental Nursing*, Blackwell Science Ltd., Oxford.

ADOLESCENTS AND
ORTHODONTIC PATIENTS

Chapter 23

Older people

LEARNING OUTCOMES

By the end of this chapter you should be able to:

1. Define who *older people* are, and state the percentage of the UK population who have some natural teeth.

2. Give reasons for oral health deterioration in older people.

3. State COMA report recommendations for the consumption of non-milk extrinsic sugars (NMES) by older people and suggest suitable alternatives in the diet.

4. List medical conditions which may prevent this group from visiting the dentist.

5. State particular dental conditions of which the group is particularly prone.

6. Describe ways of motivating patients and carers, helping them to overcome problems, including advice on denture cleaning.

WHO ARE OLDER PEOPLE?

A generation ago, nobody over 50 years in the UK would have objected to being classified as *old*.

Things have changed rapidly and dramatically over the last few decades. Diagnosis and treatment of many illnesses has vastly improved. People are living longer, eating more healthily and are keen to improve or maintain their health. Today, many people over 70 years would not consider themselves as *old*.

Until recently, in dentistry, older people were associated with being *edentulous* (having no natural teeth), or *partially dentate* (having some natural teeth), although of course both can apply to people of any age. It is now increasingly common for dental professionals to treat patients in their 80s and 90s who have natural teeth. Oral health care should be available to all, regardless of age and circumstances.

UK adult dental surveys

In the UK, adult dental surveys take place every 10 years. The 1998 survey showed that 87% of the population had some natural teeth and only 13% had full dentures[1].

The following comparison between the last two UK adult dental surveys shows that dental treatment and its uptake by the UK population have improved considerably.

1988 survey[1] – 80% of over 75 year olds had no natural teeth

1998 survey[2] – 58% of over 75 year olds had no natural teeth

British Dental Association classification of older people

The British Dental Association (BDA) describes older people as falling into three groups[3]:

1. *Entering old age.* Those who have completed careers in paid employment and/or child rearing. This is a socially constructed definition of old age including people as young as 50 years old, or from retirement age. These people are active, functionally independent and may remain so into late old age.

2. *Transitional phase.* Between a healthy, active life and frailty (*functionally dependent*). Often occurs in seventh or eighth decades but can occur at any age.

3. *Frail older people.* Vulnerable as a result of:
   - Health problems (e.g. stroke, dementia)
   - Social care needs

Of course, transition through these stages is relative, and a person may be active and independent at 85, whilst another may be frail at a much younger age.

Benefits of a healthy mouth

Benefits of a healthy mouth in the older patient include:

- Allows enjoyable eating of regular, nutritious meals (older people need more carbohydrate, less fat/protein, plenty of fibre, possibly vitamin C and D supplements).

OLDER PEOPLE

- Promotes confidence in appearance, eating and speaking in public.

- Permits clear speech.

- Prevents oral infection which may affect general health – denture wearers are prone to denture stomatitis, angular cheilitis and oral candida.

Nutrition in the older person

Healthy eating at any age is vital to good health and fitness. Changes in the following circumstances can result in poor nutrition to the older person in particular:

- Death of a spouse
- Reduction in physical activity
- Failing health or eyesight
- Illness
- Xerostomia – drug or age-related
- Deterioration of smell or taste senses
- Physical disability (unable to shop and go out)
- Poverty
- Discomfort from ill-fitting dentures
- Lack of up-to-date information on oral health and nutrition

Any of these circumstances may cause older people to skip regular, well-balanced meals and snack on easy-to-prepare alternatives which are often high in sugar. Also, many grew up in an era when adding sugar to tea and coffee was the norm and find it difficult to break this habit. Those who were young when World War II was in progress may recall that many foods were difficult to obtain. Sweet things were a rare treat and people expected to lose all their teeth by around the age of 50.

Many from this generation have full or partial dentures and they often find it difficult to change eating habits. Also, when giving oral health instruction to this group, bear in mind that they may be grandparents or great grandparents, and may need some persuasion that giving sweets to children is not such a done thing these days.

One of the recommendations of The COMA report was that the consumption of NMES should not exceed 10% of total dietary intake[4]. Special reference was made to dentate older people (over 65 years) who were advised to reduce their frequency of sugar intake.

OLDER PEOPLE

Diet

Older people generally have slightly lower energy requirements than younger adults, but still require a variety of nutritious constituents, in particular:

- Vitamin C (fruit and vegetables)
- Vitamin D (from sunlight or supplements)
- Fibre (avoiding bran-enriched products)
- Carbohydrate (pasta, rice, cereals)

They often find that they can no longer eat large meals and tend to opt for small, frequent snacks. It is obviously important that they carry on eating, but by advising on effective oral hygiene and sugar-free snack options it may be possible to reduce the risk of caries by reducing their intake of NMES in the following ways:

- Using sugar substitutes in cooking and drinks.
- Eating sugar-free sweets (some older people continually suck sweets to help dry mouths).
- Chewing sugar-free gum (if non-denture wearers).

They should, however, be made aware of the laxative effects of these products.

Barriers to dental treatment

Some older people may find it difficult to attend dental practices that are without:

- Parking facilities
- Ground-floor surgeries
- Wheelchair access
- A bus route (to the practice)

Certain common medical conditions also cause mobility problems, including:

- Angina and other heart problems
- Strokes

- Parkinson's disease

- Arthritis

- Cancer

Breaking down the barriers

The oral health educator (OHE) can help patients with poor mobility and physical impairment in the following ways:

- Suggest, or help to arrange, domiciliary visits for those who are unable to attend a practice. Try to form links with local doctors to encourage attendance.

- Check medical histories for any changes in health and consult with the dentist as necessary.

- Write brief notes on advice given so that the patients can take this home with them. Ensure names of recommended products are noted down so that patients can remember them.

- Adapt toothbrushes for patients with limited manual dexterity (e.g. handles can be enlarged for easy grip by the use of foam rubber, bicycle handlebar grips, or rubber balls). Electric toothbrushes may help and be easier to grip, but people with severe arthritis may find them difficult to switch on and too heavy.

- Demonstrate the use of *one-handed* interdental cleaning devices (i.e. bottle brushes, wood sticks, floss picks and floss handles).

- Sympathetic, understanding approach – patients will not appreciate being patronised, or treated as if they have limited mental capacity!

- Advise on the benefits of smoking cessation. It is never too late to quit, and older people with ill-health can still benefit from stopping.

- Allow extra time in the clinic (e.g. for just getting in and out of the dental chair). Think about the time of day in relation to the person being able to get up, dressed, on a bus and in for an 8.30 am appointment. Many older people may not wish to have an appointment late in the day, especially in the dark winter months.

- Some may be dependent on family members for transport or support, so always check out the needs of carers or family members and try to factor this in also.

OLDER PEOPLE

- A patient's ability to purchase and/or prepare foods may be restricted, so alternatives, which may not be good for oral health, may be chosen, particularly soft foods which can be high in NMES. Be prepared to suggest simply prepared, inexpensive meals and snacks.

- Be aware that the patient may be dependent on others (e.g. home carers), or if in residential care, may be restricted by a set menu and inadvertently have few 'healthy choices'.

- Some foods are notoriously difficult for people who wear dentures to eat (e.g. those containing seeds).

- Dentures may not fit well, due to a loss of oral muscle tone, saliva, or an impaired ability to chew or swallow (e.g. following a stroke).

- Consider the use of fluoride mouthwash or toothpaste with higher fluoride contents. Mention the availability of free toothpaste prescriptions (containing 2800 ppm or 5000 ppm of fluoride) for the people over 60s in the UK.

Oral problems of older people

Certain oral problems are commonly experienced by older people and any person with full dentures. These include:

- Xerostomia.

- Denture stomatitis.

- Angular cheilitis.

- Root caries (common in older people as recession exposes root surfaces not protected by enamel). Advise reduced sugar intake between meals, sugar-free medicines, thorough daily interdental cleaning, fluoride mouthwash, gels and toothpastes. Eating cheese to finish a meal has been shown to prevent root caries.[5]

- Sensitivity – due to recession.

- Oral cancer – more common in older people often as result of smoking/alcohol consumption. Look out for unusual red or white patches and ulcers (which do not heal). Stress the importance of annual dental examinations, even in the *edentulous*.

- Oral soft tissues, particularly the mucosa, become more fragile with ageing, and may be more prone to trauma. Reduced saliva can result in thermal trauma from hot drinks.

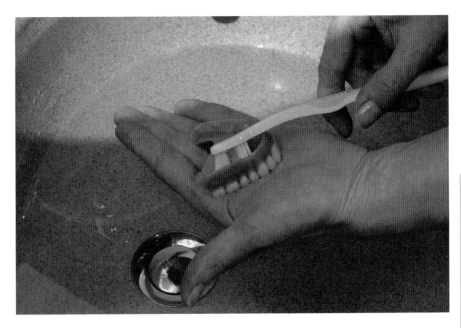

Figure 23.1 Denture cleaning (© Alison Chapman)

Denture care

As an OHE you may be asked to advise carers as well as patients on denture care.

Many people with full or partial dentures suffer problems due to ineffective denture cleaning and too-frequent soaking of dentures in bleach or well-known proprietary solutions. Older people in residential homes often have difficulty in keeping dentures clean. Carers may be untrained or frequently changed, resulting in ineffective or inconsistent denture care.

Advice to full denture wearers

Advice to older people and others who may be full denture wearers should include the following:

- Remove and clean dentures after meals (Figure 23.1) – using a soft nail brush and household soap, over a bowl or sink of water (explain the need to clean the fitting surface of a denture as well as the teeth, otherwise calculus can develop which will then need to be removed in a laboratory). If the patient has difficulty with manual dexterity, a nail brush could be wall-mounted and the denture *taken to the brush* instead. Rinse the denture after cleaning.

- Use a soft toothbrush to gently brush the soft tissues of the mouth. This ensures that no food debris is left in the mouth which could pose an aspiration risk or stagnate and contribute towards halitosis. Always check for signs of irritation or trauma.

- It is a good idea to leave dentures out at night. Be understanding that many will not wish to comply, due to embarrassment, and advise that thorough cleaning and occasionally leaving dentures out will allow oral tissues to recover. Dentures should be stored in water or left to dry (to help reduce risk of fungal re-infection).

- Many dental professionals recommend soaking dentures no more than once or twice a week (for a few minutes only) in a dilute hypochlorite solution (bactericidal/fungicidal). However, other experts[5] suggests daily soaking. Rinse in water before replacing in mouth (metal dentures are corroded by acid cleaners and should be soaked in an *alkaline peroxide solution*).

- Soaking alone will not clean dentures – they must be brushed first.

- Arrange to have dentures name-tagged when people are in residential care or nursing homes.

Advice to partial denture wearers

Advice to partial denture wearers should be the same as with full denture care, with emphasis on:

- Leaving the denture out at night
- Effective brushing/interdental cleaning of remaining teeth
- Regular dentist and hygienist appointments

Advice to carers of patients with full or partial dentures

Carers for patients with full or partial dentures (including both family and professionals) should follow these steps, when cleaning a denture or natural teeth:

1. Sit the patient comfortably in a supported-back chair, in good light. Stand behind or slightly to one side – be guided by resident's wishes. Have a mirror available.

2. Remove partial dentures (if natural teeth are to be cleaned).

3. Support head, and gently draw back lip. Use small-headed, or medium toothbrush and appropriate toothpaste. Do not use too much toothpaste.

4. Brush only two or three teeth at a time – all surfaces, taking special care with loose teeth. Any area which bleeds should be brushed more effectively.

5. If the resident tires easily, you may need to do one side of the mouth in the morning and the other side in the evening. Choose a time suitable to both.

6. Finger guards are available from shops that sell aids for disabled people if there is a concern about being bitten.

Note: OHEs may encounter patients who have had surgery for mouth cancer and wear specifically constructed appliances, known as obturators. These require specialist care, and the OHE would need advice from the patient, relatives and possibly the patient's oncology department.

Additional information for professional carers

Professional carers usually look after the oral care of residents and may find these suggestions helpful:

- An assessment of oral health should be carried out on admission and previous dental history or experience obtained where possible.
- Consider issues of cross-infection, so latex gloves should be worn.
- Residents should have their own toothbrushes and toothpaste.
- Record any observed changes in the mouth or changes reported by the resident.
- Seek further advice and support as necessary in the delivery of oral care.

Other considerations

Other considerations in the oral care of older people should include:

- Cost of treatment. This may worry the patient, and the OHE should be prepared to advise on:
  - Availability of free treatment
  - Help with dental charges for those not on benefits
  - Availability of good quality, reasonably priced, oral health aids
- Visual/hearing impairment
  - May be too proud to ask for help
  - Unable to check own mouth after cleaning
  - May not hear all instructions and advice

- Difficulty with form-filling. Be sensitive when offering help:
  - If you are completing the form ensure that you ask the patient the full question and record the full response.
  - When checking medical history, ask to see repeat prescription sheets and photocopy or scan these into the notes.

Remember! Older people were once as young and fit as you (and may still be, or even more so). Although sometimes frail, they are still intelligent and should be treated with the same respect that you give to all patients.

SELF-ASSESSMENT

1. Assume that you have been asked to give a talk to a small group of carers in a residential home for older people, write short notes about background information required and how you would prepare for the session (include structure and content of the talk).
2. Write short notes on the care of full and partial dentures.

REFERENCES

1. Office of Population Censuses and Surveys (1991) *Adult Dental Health Survey (1988).* HMSO, London.
2. Office for National Statistics (2000) *Adult Dental Health Survey (1998): Oral Health in the United Kingdom, 1998.* Stationery Office Books, London.
3. British Dental Association (2003), *Oral Healthcare for Older People: 2020 Vision,* British Dental Association, London.
4. Health Education Authority (1999) *Sugars in the Diet.* Health Education Authority, London.
5. Papas, A.S., Joshi, A., Belanger, A.J., Kent, R.L., Palmer, C.A., Defaola, P.F. (1995) Dietary models for root caries, *American Journal of Clinical Nutrition,* 61, 417–422, American Society for Clinical Nutrition.

Chapter 24

At risk and special care patients

LEARNING OUTCOMES

By the end of this chapter you should be able to:

1. List patients considered to be at a higher risk than average of developing dental disease.

2. Explain circumstances associated with these patients which increase their risks of developing dental disease.

3. Be aware of the changes to the recommendation of pre-treatment antibiotics.

4. State how the oral health educator (OHE) can assist *at risk* and *special care* patients.

WHO ARE 'AT RISK' PATIENTS?

When talking about *at risk* patients in the context of giving OHE, we mean people who, through no fault of their own, are at higher risk than the general population of developing dental disease, or find it difficult to manage oral health procedures.

Patients in this group include special care patients covered in certain target groups: pregnant women, orthodontic/obturator appliance wearers, and older people. Some of these patients fit into more than one category, for example:

- Medically compromised patients (those with chronic, systemic disease).

- People with physical impairment.

- People with learning disabilities and phobias.

- People of low socioeconomic status (including homeless and recreational drug users).

- People who never visit the dentist unless in pain.

- Patients with dental phobia.

- Severely compromised patients.

Medically compromised patients

Medically compromised patients include people with diabetes, epilepsy, haemophilia and those on continual medication. Historically, patients with heart valve defects who were prescribed antibiotics prior to treatment to prevent infective endocarditis, were treated as medically compromised.

However, the BNF British National Formulary[2] (BNF) editors and clinical advisers have reviewed the NICE guidelines on Antimicrobial Prophylaxis Against infective endocarditis in Adults and Children Undergoing Interventional Procedures (March 2008). BNF 55 (section 5.1) reflects these radical guidelines and advises that antimicrobial prophylaxis is no longer recommended for the prevention of endocarditis in patients undergoing dental and non-dental procedures. Prophylaxis may expose patients to the adverse effects of antimicrobials when the evidence of benefit has not been proven.

Medical defence unions have advised that anyone found to prescribe antibiotic prophylaxis, even if the patient requests it, will be liable for any adverse reaction.

Patients with diabetes

Patients with poorly controlled diabetes are more prone to periodontal disease (due to vascular deficiencies and a relatively lower immune response). They may find cooperation with the OHE difficult to sustain. It is important for the OHE to observe these guidelines:

- Keep to time with appointments, as the patient may have to eat at regular intervals to avoid *hypoglycaemia*. Children needing to snack on chocolate bars, etc., may be more prone to caries.

- Be vigilant for signs of impending coma (the patient may become confused or irritable).

Patients with epilepsy

Some epileptic patients have their condition well-controlled by drug therapy, others less so. A sympathetic and tactful approach is necessary as certain patients may be sensitive about the stigma attached to this condition.

Patients may require encouragement to keep regular dental/hygiene appointments because they need excellent plaque control. They may have *gingival overgrowth* associated with taking anticonvulsant drugs, e.g. *Phenytoin*. Plaque aggravates this drug-related condition.

Patients with haemophilia (and other bleeding disorders)

With modern treatments, these conditions are usually well-controlled, but unnecessary risks which may lead to blood loss need to be avoided.

Dental procedures (i.e. injections) may put haemophiliacs at risk of haemorrhaging, and it is therefore advisable to establish good oral health in childhood so that minimal dental intervention is necessary.

Patients on continual prescription medication

Patients taking many different medications simultaneously may find it difficult to adhere to an oral health regimen because of how the drugs need to be taken (e.g. with food, after food, early morning, or last thing at night). Some drugs may have side effects such as nausea and vomiting, which can lead to dehydration and *xerostomia*.

Patients with physical impairment

Patients with physical impairment include:

- Mobility impairment (from birth, illness or an accident).
- Limited manual dexterity (e.g. arthritis, stroke, Parkinson's disease, multiple sclerosis).
- Hearing impairment.
- Visual impairment.

Patients with mental impairment

Patients with mental impairment include:

- Learning disabilities, which may be due to a range of conditions such as Down's syndrome, autism and associated disorders, head injuries, dyslexia, dementia and emotional disorders such as depression.
- Inappropriate/challenging behaviour.
- Short attention span.
- Phobia (sometimes dental phobia).

All patients in these physical and mental 'impairment groups' require time and patience as well as tact and special arrangements (where possible) when they attend for dental treatment. Some may need to be treated in special clinics

Table 24.1 Acceptable and unacceptable phrases for certain special care patients

Acceptable phrases	Unacceptable phrases
Wheelchair user	Wheelchair bound
Person with epilepsy	Suffers from epilepsy
Person with disabilities	Handicapped person
Hearing/speech impaired	Deaf/dumb
Accessible toilet	Disabled toilet

or in their own homes by a community dental team. Those who can attend the surgery may need help with access for wheelchairs and specially adapted oral hygiene aids, such as toothbrushes with larger handles for easier grip, and help to fill in forms if visually or hearing impaired.

The patient's own capabilities must be considered and the OHE must assess if an individual has the physical and cognitive ability to:

- Carry out effective personal oral care

- Communicate needs to others

- Access dental services

- Make healthy, informed choices regarding diet

Phrases used for special care patients

Table 24.1 shows acceptable and unacceptable phrases for certain special care patients (F. Marriott, personal communication).

People of low socioeconomic status

OHEs working in hospitals, the community dental service and *drop in centres* are more likely to help these patients (which include the homeless and recreational drug users) than those working in private practice.

Tact, understanding and kindness are needed when helping homeless people. Remember that many patients have not always been in these circumstances. They often only request emergency treatment and will not attend again, thereby missing the opportunity for the OHE to provide further assistance. Homeless patients and those living in poverty may also find it impossible to afford oral hygiene aids, so it is a good idea to have free samples available to give out. Commercial companies may be able to help supply these, although, if the patient living on the streets they may have no facilities to carry out oral health

AT RISK AND SPECIAL CARE PATIENTS

procedures such as running water and sinks. A tactful, empathetic approach may be the key to persuading them to return for further treatment.

This group may also include people who are taking recreational drugs, who may exhibit challenging behaviour due to drug addiction. The OHE should be familiar with the signs of drug and solvent addiction and knowledge of drugs, their effects and substitutes such as *methadone*, which is cariogenic.

Once again, great tact is needed. The OHE may require special training (usually available for those working in the community), and must be prepared to adapt advice according to patients' lifestyles and capabilities.

Patients with dental phobia

Patients with extreme phobia are also more likely to be encountered in a hospital or a community dentistry setting, since they would have been referred by dentists who have no time to cope with their special needs in the practice. The OHE must be guided by the instructions of the dentist, but can do much to help patients with phobia by a gentle, understanding approach.

It is important to conduct oral hygiene sessions in a 'non-dental' setting, free from *dental equipment noises* and disinfectant smells. It may be appropriate for the OHE not to wear a uniform (which can be a barrier), and to talk to the patient in comfortable surroundings. Much time and patience is needed and a sympathetic questioning technique employed in order to ascertain the source and causes of their phobia. It may take a number of visits before the patient is comfortable enough to look at oral hygiene aids and discuss any treatment which may be required, but achieving a positive result can give the educator great job satisfaction.

Severely compromised patients

Generally, patients whose needs render them severely compromised live in specialised, residential homes, although some are able to live in their own homes with family members providing care. They include:

- Paraplegics (from birth or accidents)
- Patients with motor-neurone disease
- Patients with dementia
- Patients needing palliative care

An OHE may be asked to give talks to carers about establishing and maintaining dental care for these patients. It is wise to find out exactly what is required before giving such a talk to find out who the audience is and what procedures are currently being adopted. If you are required to give specific advice for individual patients, the patient will need to be seen by a dentist and an oral health care plan set-up. Home-carers often have a difficult time and also need empathy, support and advice.

Be prepared to advise on:

- Positioning the patient for effective and comfortable mouth care, including safety of patient and carer.

- Safe, effective plaque control.

- Adaptation of oral hygiene aids.

- Preserving the dignity of the patients and encouraging them to do as much as possible for themselves.

Remember! All these groups require extra care, consideration, help, respect and encouragement with oral health procedures. Treat patients as your equal (because they are). Communicate appropriately. If the patient agrees, carers should be included in the conversation but your main point of focus should be the patient.

SELF-ASSESSMENT

1. Define *at risk* patients.

2. List from memory, patients you would include as being *at risk* from dental problems, and in undergoing treatment.

3. What do you understand by the term *medically compromised* in relation to dental treatment?

4. In brief sentences, describe what problems the following groups may encounter (in relation to dentistry):

   - Patients who are diabetics

   - Patients with epilepsy

   - Patients with haemophilia

   - Patients on continual medication

   - Patients with any medical condition (e.g. physical impairment).

   - Homeless patients and recreational drug users

   - Patients with dental phobia

5. How can you as an OHE help in the treatment of *at risk* patients?

6. Write short notes on:

   – The reasons people give for not visiting the dentist

   – Poverty and oral health

   – Medically compromised patients

REFERENCES

1. British Dental Association, British Medical Association and Royal Pharmaceutical Society of Great Britain (1998) *Dental Practitioners' Formulary 1998–2000 (incorporating British National Formulary 36)*. British Dental Association, British Medical Association and Royal Pharmaceutical Society of Great Britain, London.
2. BNF 55, British National Formulary, March 2008 (2008). Available at www.bnf.org, accessed 21 March 2008.

AT RISK AND SPECIAL CARE PATIENTS

Chapter 25

Minority ethnic populations in the UK

LEARNING OUTCOMES

By the end of this chapter you should be able to:

1. State the percentage of the UK population represented by minority ethnic groups.
2. List the barriers to the uptake of dental treatment by these patients.
3. Describe ways of breaking down these barriers.
4. List guidelines for producing suitable promotional material for this target group.

INTRODUCTION

Oral health educators (OHEs) are almost certain to give oral health education to patients from minority ethnic groups. It is therefore important to have some knowledge of the ideas and beliefs commonly encountered in people of these groups.

The UK 2001 census[1] revealed that 7.85% of the UK population is made up of black and minority ethnic groups. Taking England separately, the percentage of people from minority ethnic groups increased from 6 to 9% in the decade proceeding the 1991 census[2]. Older members of this population (particularly Caribbean) may have migrated here in the 1950s, but an increasingly large proportion are born in the UK.

Since the 2001 census, with more European countries joining the European Community, many citizens have migrated to the UK. People from the European Community are likely to feature more and more in the work of the OHE in future years. It is possible that their command of the English language is limited, and so it is important to know how to source information in their languages where possible.

BARRIERS TO DENTAL TREATMENT

Whilst it would be wrong to generalise, health and community personnel who work with minority ethnic groups are aware that the uptake of dental treatment in this section of the population is well below average. There are a number of reasons for this, including:

- Older generations – may have never seen a dentist and may not see the need to take their children, or commonly only attend when they have a problem as they would in their country of birth.

- Bad experiences in country of origin – may have caused distress and reluctance to visit the dentist.

- Conflicting views in the family – concerning the importance of oral health.

- Lack of awareness of services and facilities.

- Communication can be difficult – if no interpreter is available.

- Problems with a male dentist treating women – certain religions (e.g. orthodox Muslims) must not allow a man other than a husband to see them unveiled.

BREAKING DOWN THE BARRIERS

The OHE has a unique opportunity to break down some of these barriers in the following ways:

- Meet with community leaders – find out what help is needed to encourage regular dental attendance.

- Contact doctors, health visitors, practice nurses and teachers who may already be involved with a health programme in the area. Oral health is a part of general health and it may be possible to join forces with other health professionals in giving advice on:

  – Diet/nutrition – advice is often welcomed, but consult health visitors/school teachers first. For example: the Muslim faith forbids the eating of pig and carnivorous animals.
      OHEs in areas with a high percentage of ethnic groups will need to be aware of the timing of religious festivals that involve fasting, such as *Diwali* (Hindu) and *Ramadan* (Muslim).

MINORITY ETHNIC POPULATIONS IN THE UK

Heavily spiced foods can contribute to staining of the dentition and there may be issues with abrasion. Find out what is in snack/drink items that are being consumed. Remember that lacto-vegetarian or vegan (no animal products at all) regimes may be adhered to by any nationality.

– Betel nut chewing (a carcinogenic habit in certain Eastern cultures) – produces a red stain. It is used to relieve stress, similar to tobacco.

– Check that sugar/food is not being put in babies' bottles.

– Think about oral health products you recommend. Some may not be suitable for use by certain cultures. For example: certain saliva substitutes contain *porcine* (pig) *mucin*, and certain mouthwashes contain alcohol.

– Find out how to address people – different cultures adopt a different format for names.

– Smoking – the NHS provides leaflets in other languages.

GUIDELINES FOR PROMOTIONAL MATERIAL

When producing resources, bear in mind that each minority group has its own culture, traditions and customs. One leaflet will not be appropriate for all and the OHE should bear in mind the following points when producing material:

- Individuals in an illustration – should reflect the ethnicity, customs and culture of the target group.

- Written material should have the appropriate language. For example: Punjabi can be written using two different alphabets, depending on the country of origin.

- Pictures of foodstuffs – should relate to the culture and include appropriate, traditional foods/labels.

- Pictures of people eating – must reflect the fact that some religions would regard it as offensive to eat with the left hand.

- Certain symbols and icons – not universally recognised. For example: some cultures reverse the meaning of a tick or a cross on a questionnaire.

- Some cultures read *right to left* or use picture language.

- Handouts/leaflets – should be presented with clear, good quality print/readability.

- Pilot material with a community leader before distribution.

It is possible to find dental leaflets translated into a number of Asian languages and Chinese. With the arrival of many groups from European countries, it is becoming necessary to produce material in their languages, so ask about the availability of these also.

SELF-ASSESSMENT

1. What percentage of the population did the 2001 survey show came from black and other minority ethnic groups?

2. List the reasons why the uptake of dental treatment is poor amongst ethnic minorities.

3. Write a paragraph explaining how you, as an OHE, can help to overcome barriers to dental treatment in this target group.

4. How would you obtain leaflets in appropriate languages to use as resources?

5. In designing a leaflet for a specific ethnic group, what points would you consider?

REFERENCES

1. Office for National Statistics (2003) *2001 UK Census of Population*. The Stationery Office, London.
2. Office of Population, Censuses and Surveys (1993) *1991 UK Census of Population*. HMSO, London.

MINORITY ETHNIC POPULATIONS IN THE UK

Chapter 26
Other health professionals

LEARNING OUTCOMES

By the end of this chapter you should be able to:

1. List other health professionals who may be giving oral health advice to the public.

2. Confidently pass on your knowledge of oral health to these professionals who may be patients themselves, or who may be passing on advice to patients or students.

3. Suggest appropriate sources of oral health information and resources for this group.

INTRODUCTION

Although UK surveys[1,2] show that the oral health of the nation is improving generally, poor oral health and ignorance of positive health choices are still widespread in certain social groups. An oral health educator (OHE) has a vital role to play in improving oral health awareness amongst these groups. This includes keeping up to date with annual events (national and local) such as *National No Smoking Day* (each March) and the British Dental Health Foundation's *National Smile Month* (each May).

Such events are great opportunities to deliver information to a community and for the OHE to become involved with other people who provide oral health education: by setting up a display or an exhibition within a general theme, such as a 'cardiac roadshow', or to give a talk to an antenatal or postnatal group, or to parents at a school parents' evening.

WHO ELSE PROVIDES ORAL HEALTH EDUCATION?

Health professionals in a number of different sectors give oral health advice to the public. These professionals include:

- Health visitors

- Community and hospital midwives

- Social workers

- Community/school nurses

- Doctors and practice nurses

- Hospital nursing teams (in-patients)

- Rehabilitation teams, i.e. multidisciplinary teams (MDT) which can include physiotherapists, occupational therapists, speech and language therapists

- Carers

- Dieticians

- Pharmacists

- Teachers – as forms part of the National Curriculum

- Nursery leaders

- Commercial organisations (companies selling oral health aids, etc.)

- Health reporters in magazines/newspapers

Remember! It is very important that all providers give the same messages to avoid confusion and conflicting advice among recipients. For example: midwives, health visitors and school nurses in the UK were advising parents to use baby foods and drinks which the dental profession knew to be cariogenic. As a result, the Health Education Authority (now the Health Development Agency) produced a useful training manual[3] for health visitors and school nurses.

The OHE should be aware of how professionals obtain other information to pass on to patients, and may be able to put them in contact with representatives of large dental companies who will usually be helpful in providing them with leaflets and sometimes free samples. Some companies produce project material for use with schoolchildren, and it is worth asking dental representatives if anything like this is available for teachers who may be OHE patients. Information may also be sourced from leaflets in hospitals and health centres.

OTHER HEALTH PROFESSIONALS

GAINING CONFIDENCE TO DELIVER ADVICE TO OTHER PROFESSIONALS

Taking part in community projects is a good way of helping to build up confidence in delivering oral health education to groups. OHEs will learn a lot by listening to the people they are working with in such projects, and the education process is therefore two-way.

GIVING ADVICE TO INDIVIDUAL HEALTH EDUCATION PROFESSIONALS

Careful lesson planning is vital, and should take into account the patient's profession. For example: if the patient is a dental professional, OHEs know that they can use dental terms. If the patient is, for example, a dietician who will not necessarily understand technical dental jargon, OHEs should plan the lesson accordingly, perhaps asking the subject's opinion regarding dietary advice for patients.

Use appropriate resources. It is assumed, for example, that because a patient is well educated and working in a health-related field, they will be aware of the importance of the benefits of fluoride or interdental cleaning. This is not always the case and often considerable tact is necessary in finding out what dental aids patients use and in persuading them that change might be helpful. An appropriate evaluation of each session should be undertaken.

Remember! Most patients will see the OHE in a role of someone the dentist has suggested can help them, but other health professionals could see it as insulting that the dentist feels that their oral hygiene could be improved. A good initial approach with such patients can be to ask how they feel about their current oral hygiene or dietary habits and whether they feel change will be beneficial.

Having mastered the art of dealing with other health professionals, OHEs will find themselves less nervous in giving advice to the general public and usually find that the same respectful, yet confident approach works well with everyone, even children!

SELF-ASSESSMENT

1. List at least 10 health professionals who may be involved in delivering oral health advice to the public.

2. What is the most important point to remember for all health professionals giving advice on oral health?

3. Write short notes about sources of information on OHE which you can recommend to other health professionals.

4. In setting up an exhibition for other health professionals, how might your material differ from that produced for members of the general public?

OTHER HEALTH PROFESSIONALS

5. List three ways in which you can increase your confidence in talking to other health professionals.

6. Write short notes on the points to remember when talking to health professionals about their own oral health.

REFERENCES

1. Office for National Statistics (2000) *Adult Dental Health Survey (1998): Oral Health in the United Kingdom, 1998*. Stationery Office Books, London.
2. Office for National Statistics (2004) *2003 Dental Health Survey of Children and Young People*. Stationery Office Books, London.
3. Health Education Authority (1996) *A Handbook for Dental Health for Health Visitors and School Nurses*, 4th edn. Health Education Authority, London.

OTHER HEALTH PROFESSIONALS

Chapter 27

Planning education case studies

LEARNING OUTCOMES

By the end of this chapter you should be able to:

1. Set up a record of experience.

2. Acquire confidence to carry out case studies.

3. Have the knowledge to set up an exhibition or display (in conjunction with Chapter 17).

RECORD OF EXPERIENCE

This chapter is particularly aimed at NEBDN students and should be read in conjunction with the NEBDN exam pack.

Part A of the *record of experience* concerns giving oral health education to 10 individuals from different target groups. There is a variety of topics to choose from, ranging from advice to parents of toddlers, to care of dentures in older people.

Details of each education session must be recorded on a *log sheet tracker*, each patient must be seen at least twice, and the topic of the visit recorded. Log sheet records explain how you planned and evaluated sessions, and how the patient reacted.

Getting started

It is a good idea to ask for sufficient notice from your dentist before seeing a patient, in order to study their dental record and plan the session effectively. Having studied the patient's records and found what is required, the guidelines given in Chapter 17 should be followed.

It is normal to feel nervous and apprehensive about talking to a patient, particularly if somebody else in the workplace is observing. However, once you have talked to the person, found out a little about them and planned what steps are required, the second visit or patient will not nearly be as intimidating. Remember that the patient may be more nervous than you.

Greet patients warmly, introducing yourself with a smile, and invite them to remove outdoor clothing and take a seat (preferably in a comfortable chair in a setting free of dental equipment, noises and smells). However, this is not always possible – most hygienists and therapists carry out their sessions whilst they work clinically or immediately afterwards, often with the patient in the dental chair. It is the educator's attitude, body language and knowledge that puts the patient at ease and helps achieve the desired results.

Do not expect an instant change of attitude or behaviour in patients. It often takes years of getting to know them (and what goes on in their lives), before they are persuaded to change their behaviour. Obviously you do not have years, so you have to do the best you can in two or three encounters. Therefore, be meticulous in obtaining as much background information as you can (you may know a lot about the patients already if they are regular attenders at the practice), which can be used in the opening greeting.

For example:

Hello, Mrs Jones, we have met several times when Mr Smith has been treating your children. My name is Ann and Mr Smith has asked me to discuss little Freddy's diet with you as he has already had two fillings. By the way, how is Freddy enjoying his new playgroup? I remember you telling Mr Smith that he was apprehensive about starting there.

In that way, you have begun a relationship with Mrs Jones, impressed her by remembering her conversation with the dentist and given her a chance to chat about something other than Freddy's diet (may be relevant to his caries record), which will help to put her at her ease. It is a good idea to keep a notebook with you and jot down points like Freddy's playgroup (but not anything you perceive as confidential between patient and dentist).

If it is likely that the dentist is going to refer a patient to you at the time of examination, make a few relevant notes in the notebook then, which can become part of your record of experience (although when submitting to examiners do not include anything which would identify the patient).

You will soon find that talking to patients is much easier than you imagined and probably one of the most rewarding aspects of the OHE's job.

Difficult patients

Of course there are always difficult patients who will grumble about everything and some are even openly hostile. Often aggressive behaviour is a 'cover-up' for anxiety or fear. If you tell yourself that aggressive behaviour is concealing something in the patient's life that you do not know about and treat them with extra kindness and patience, more often than not they will respond positively.

Teenagers can be particularly challenging – often they will refuse eye contact and it is difficult to establish a relationship with somebody who behaves in this way. Once again, tact and patience may achieve results – seeing the teenager without a parent can help (you can always ask the patient's permission to include mum or dad at the end of the session to briefly explain the points you have made).

It may help if you can find some common ground upon which to approach the teenager. Girls of this age are very concerned about their appearance and you can liken care of their teeth and time spent to the meticulous way in which make-up is applied. Teenage boys are often more interested in sport. Once again *background information* might enable you to get your point over. For example: 'Have you noticed (name of sporting hero's) stunning smile? Wouldn't it be gross to see red, swollen gums and blackened teeth when he's interviewed on TV?' You could even have posters of sports or other personalities in the PDU, showing their beautifully cared-for teeth.

Completing the log sheet

After each session, you will be required to complete the NEBDN log sheet, which must be signed by a *supervising witness* (i.e. a dentist). The witness does not need to be present during the session, but should be aware (through prior discussion) of your proposal, and approved your lesson plan. You can have the witness present if you wish, or someone else dentally qualified who will report back to them (i.e. a hygienist, therapist, practice manager, nurse or your tutor). You must inform the dentist about how the session went and discuss any points of concern before asking them to sign the record.

Expanded case studies

Part B of the record of experience involves the completion of two *expanded case studies*. It is likely (but not mandatory) that you will choose these from the 10 patients referred to you by the dentist.

Carrying out two detailed studies requires much thought, input and dedication. However, case studies are quite personal and you will get to know your patient extremely well. If you throw yourself into each, you can become an important catalyst in changing patients' oral health régimes.

Patients who require a fair amount of help and encouragement (and who will keep appointments) should be chosen – advice from your dentist or hygienist may help you make this decision. One patient must be an adult and one a child or adolescent.

Therefore, when deciding on which case studies to expand upon, try to choose patients who are keen to improve their oral health, and who have either:

1. A number of things to achieve in order to improve oral hygiene, or

2. A special reason for improving oral hygiene.

Case study examples

Here are two examples of expanded case studies undertaken by former students.

1. The patient with a number of things to improve

   A 47-year-old lady had extensive complex restorations, in other words, large fillings (many of them old and worn but better not replaced), crowns and bridges. Despite trying hard to improve her standard of oral health, she could not achieve effective plaque control; consequently her gingival condition was poor and deteriorating.

   One student saw her about six times, got to know her lifestyle and fired her with enthusiasm to improve her oral health. Under this guidance, the patient learned to floss effectively, used interdental brushes and performed efficient plaque removal from heavily filled teeth using a rechargeable electric toothbrush.

   Both the OHE and her patient gained a great deal of satisfaction from the exercise and the examiners liked the way she had tackled and explained her case study.

2. The patient with a special reason for improving oral health
   Another student had a 15-year-old relative who was a patient at her practice, and who came into the category of *special care*. He had moderate learning difficulties and in her words: 'was about 9–11 years old in understanding and capability – but keen to improve'.

The OHE, acting upon her dentist's instructions, decided that she would try to improve:

- His toothbrushing, which left much to be desired, resulting in a poor gingival condition.

- His diet. He consumed numerous high-sugar snacks and drinks between meals, resulting in a high caries rate.

PLANNING EDUCATION CASE STUDIES

The OHE tackled both these aspects, which in ordinary circumstances would probably have been too much. It is often better to tackle one aspect of oral health at a time.

However, in this case, she had frequent access to the patient who cooperated and enjoyed the sessions. The OHE made large mouth models to demonstrate effective toothbrushing and helped him perform brushing techniques in front of a mirror. She also showed him how to use disclosing tablets and encouraged him with 'before and after' photographs of his mouth.

When his brushing had improved, she taught him to look at the labels on his snacks. When the time came to submit her case study, she was still working with him, and recognised how much more time was needed. However, she learned a great deal about working with such a patient and was able to explain this in her write-up.

Arranging appointments

After selecting two patients for expanded studies, the next step is to arrange several appointments in advance, making sure that you have allowed around 30 min for an adult patient. For children, you may need slightly more or less time depending upon the age of the child and the problems to be tackled. Remember that children (particularly under school age) have a short attention span.

Case study report

After each session make notes of everything that happened in order to write a report of 2000 words at the end of the study. If appropriate, you can include photographs, although they are not essential and candidates who do not include them do not lose marks.

Try to use imagination as well as knowledge in producing the report, which must demonstrate that you have a good depth of knowledge about the topic you have chosen and about the messages you are giving[1]. Write it out in rough first, and follow style guidelines from the exam pack. This rough copy can be seen by your tutor, who can make suggestions to help you improve it and it can also become your spare copy to refer to when your finished report has been submitted for assessment.

Exhibition or display

Part C of the current exam format is concerned with designing either a display or an exhibition.

This will probably be carried out in your workplace. However, not all dentists are cooperative and some practices simply do not have the space. In the past, students have set up exhibitions for carers in residential homes, schools, hospitals, clinics and church halls.

Reasons for a choice of topic may be that either:

1. Your dentist or hygienist has noticed some aspect of patients' oral health which requires improvement. This can be targeted in your practice.

2. You or your dentist is asked by friends who are teachers or health professionals to improve oral health knowledge with their class or patients. This is usually done outside the workplace.

You will have received a *proforma* for the exhibition or display in the exam pack which makes planning considerably easier.

How to set up an exhibition is covered in Chapter 17, and there now follows some guidance notes on choosing a topic for your exhibition or display.

Choosing a topic

Try to choose a topic which is relevant to the practice or workplace.

Maybe your dentist has strong feelings that all patients should floss regularly, but they or the hygienist has noticed that responses to their suggestions have not been good. This would be your chance to mount an exhibition on the topic, acquiring knowledge on the subject to educate patients and collect resources from company representatives and others.

The exhibition or display must be self-explanatory, since you are not expected to be there to answer patients' questions. Wherever it is held, it can probably be left up for a while. If it is not to be held in the workplace you can be guided by the requirements of the person who has asked you to set it up.

Examples of exhibitions/displays

Here are several examples of exhibitions/displays by former students.

1. In response to a request from a teacher who was a patient at her practice, an OHE set up an exhibition on 'Tooth-friendly Packed Lunches' in a local primary school. The children came in a class at a time in their lunch hours and the OHE stayed with her exhibition and answered questions from children and staff.

2. A student, whose teenagers were in a swimming club, noticed that young swimmers, many of whom were patients at her practice, continually sipped

fizzy drinks whilst waiting for races. Her dentist had noticed a surprising rise in teenage erosion so she set up an exhibition on the subject and took it to the local secondary school.

3. Another student set up an exhibition on healthy snacks in a local nursery school. The staff had noticed that some of the children had diets high in sugar and their dentist became aware of caries in a number of nursery school children.

The possibilities are endless, but it is a good idea to pick a topic on which you and your dentist agree and in which you have a particular interest. If you are interested in your topic, your enthusiasm will carry you along and will be evident to examiners.

Exhibition plan

Having decided upon the subject of your exhibition, you need to make a campaign plan, enlisting the help of your dentist and other members of staff, if possible. For example:

1. What are my aims and objectives?
2. Venue – where shall I set it up?
3. When would be a good time to do it?
4. Who is the target group?
5. What resources should I use?

Your tutors will assist you in all aspects of planning and setting up an exhibition or display and you can also follow the guidelines in the exam pack. You need to include a method (e.g. a questionnaire) so that you can briefly describe the outcome of your exhibition on the record sheet. There is only room to write brief notes on this sheet, and so your outcome evaluation might be something like this:

Following my exhibition, 25 patients demonstrated that they could use dental floss effectively; 20 patients said that they would try to use floss regularly; 4 patients would try to use another interdental method, and 1 patient would not change their behaviour.

Although the current format does not require OHEs to remain with an exhibition for a day, by doing so you can assess what patients have learned.

SELF-ASSESSMENT

Planning an expanded case study.

Think of a patient with whom an expanded case study would be suitable (an existing patient or an acquaintance), and write a plan on the basis of the following points:

- Report title – think of a short, catchy, relevant title that will have examiners wanting to read on.

- Introduction – a brief paragraph, introducing yourself and where you work (could be accompanied by a photograph).

- Reason for choosing patients – who are they, reasons for choice? If possible, include a personal/practice reason and a scientifically based reason. For example: 'My dentist had noticed an increase in the number of teenage children presenting with erosion and the 2003 Survey of Child Dental Health gives statistics to support this'.

- Write aim(s) and objectives – three objectives is a good number. Too many objectives will complicate the project. Avoid using words such as *know* and *understand*. Use words like *demonstrate, explain, describe, choose* and *recognise*.

- Method – explain what you plan to do and where and how you will do it. How long will it take? How many visits will it involve? Do you need to involve other staff members?

- Results – what happened (statistically)? For example: 'After four sessions, my patient has stopped sipping fizzy drinks; limiting them to once a day at mealtimes and is trying to embrace a less-acidic diet'. These results need to be collated on paper to show examiners (e.g. graphs or pie charts).

- Assessment – how will you prove that your patient has acquired new knowledge and skills?

Will you:

– Design a questionnaire? If so, will you need to pilot it, and with whom?
– Arrange for the patient(s) to demonstrate new skills? (You will need photos or another method of showing the examiners what happened.)
– Plan a follow-up visit at a later date?
– Give patient(s) a target (e.g. change to an acidic-drink-free diet)?
– Arrange for your dentist or hygienist to monitor patients' long-term improvements (you will need a method of assessing this)?

- Evaluation. Did your study achieve your objectives, and if not, why? Did you encounter any particular problems? If so, how would you do things differently next time?

- Finishing touches. These can make all the difference to the presentation:

– If possible have the title (simply and attractively displayed) on the cover.
– Include a contents page (to help the examiners find their way around).

- Keep explanations simple and to the point (remember the examiners have to read many reports).
- Pay attention to grammar, spelling and punctuation.
- Keep to around the permitted 2000 words. Other relevant material can be put in an appendix (which is not included in the word count).
- If including photographs, use a maximum of three or four. These should be clear and show relevant details.
- If you wish, you can thank relevant people for their help in an acknowledgements page.

REFERENCE

1. Levine, R.S., Stillman-Lowe, C.R. (2004) *The Scientific Basis of Oral Health Education*. BDJ Books, London.

SECTION 6
ORAL HEALTH AND SOCIETY

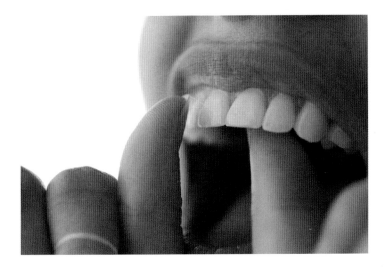

INTRODUCTION

This section looks at how UK society is working to improve the oral health of the nation in the twenty-first century.

It examines the issues of *socialisation* (i.e. the impact that oral health education has upon family and other social groups), and *epidemiology* – the study of the incidence of disease and distribution within the population.

It also looks at *evidence-based prevention* (i.e. advice based on research-based, written evidence), and different levels of prevention according to patient need are discussed. Quality control in dental services and the ways in which dental treatment can currently be obtained in the UK are also addressed.

The section concludes with a chapter setting out the differences and similarities between oral health promotion and education, and explains how the two interrelate and work together to improve the oral health of the population in the twenty-first century.

Chapter 28
Sociology

LEARNING OUTCOMES

By the end of this chapter you should be able to:

1. Define *sociology* and *socialisation* and explain factors that influence individual behaviour in the uptake of health care.

2. Define and differentiate between *primary* and *secondary* socialisation.

3. Explain what is meant by *values* and *norms*.

4. Show awareness of the UK *Office for National Statistics' Register* of *Social Groups* and give examples of *social class differences* within the population.

5. Explain what is meant by the *iceberg effect, victim blaming* and the *performance gap*.

SOCIOLOGY

Sociology can be defined as *the study of the structure and functioning of human society.*

In order to understand the uptake of dental treatment by the UK population, the oral health educator (OHE) needs to study the way society functions in the twenty-first century.

Sociologists tell us that individual behaviour in the uptake of health care is influenced by[1]:

1. Political decisions. For example: UK government funding changes to NHS Dentistry in 1990 resulted in many dentists entering the private sector. Consequently, many people marginally above the social benefits line can no longer afford to attend the dentist.

2. Cultural influences. For example: certain immigrant sections of society, particularly the older generation who have not always lived in the UK, were not brought up to attend the dentist unless they experience pain.

SOCIALISATION

Socialisation is the process by which infants and young children become aware of society and their relationships with others[2]. From the moment of birth an infant begins the learning process. For example: in these early days parents talk to babies, smile at them and very soon the baby responds and imitates smiles and sounds. Thus begins the process of *socialisation*.

The OHE needs to understand the two main stages of socialisation. These are:

1. *Primary socialisation.* Describes learning that takes place in preschool years beginning as soon as the child is born. Many sociologists think that beliefs and attitudes learned in these years are almost impossible to change in later life. This is when a child is very receptive to learning about topics such as toothbrushing and a healthy diet, and the *values* and *norms* of family life and behaviour. The child learns from:

   - Parents.

   - Close family members (grandparents and siblings) – about how to behave within the family. This learning is vital to establish healthy behaviour patterns. Children deprived of these early learning opportunities often grow up with behavioural problems.

   - The reconstituted family – many families are involved in relationship breakdown and repair, which can have a profound effect upon primary socialisation, with a child's learning being interrupted or changed.

2. *Secondary socialisation* – refers to learning that takes place outside of the close family. This is usually when the child begins preschool or primary school and is influenced by the ideas and practices of:

   - Teachers

   - Peers

   - Media

   - Carers

   - Health care professionals (including the dental team)

Secondary socialisation provided by teachers and other professionals is referred to as *formal secondary socialisation*, and that learned from peers or the media known as *informal secondary socialisation*. During these educational years the child should hopefully learn to behave acceptably outside the home (i.e. the *values and norms* of society).

SOCIOLOGY

Values

The values of society are also referred to as *collected beliefs* (e.g. 'society demands equality in health care for all individuals'). These are *ideals* and OHEs soon become aware that there is not equality in many aspects of dental treatment.

Norms

Norms describe the most common patterns of behaviour – but not everyone conforms to these patterns. It could be said that it is the *norm* for people to brush their teeth twice daily or the *norm* to have regular six-monthly dental check-ups.

In UK society, there is still a social divide between the *professional* and *working* classes, which dates back to Victorian times when there were *upper classes* (employers and gentry) and *lower classes* (who worked for them). In modern UK society, a person can be classified according to their *socioeconomic* status.

Table 28.1 shows the UK National Statistics Socioeconomic Classification (NS-SEC) of analytical classes[3].

These social classes are not simple to analyse, and are designed principally for the purpose of epidemiological surveys. Surveys[4] reveal that social class reflects values, norms and beliefs held by different community groups – these social factors influence behaviour.

Epidemiological studies and surveys[4] also show that people from the higher social classes are generally, though not always, the most 'future orientated' (i.e. more likely to take preventive action and visit the dentist more often). They also have the lowest refined carbohydrate intake. Predictably, adolescents from families in the lower social classes are more likely to snack on sugary items and these families have higher caries rates and visit the dentist irregularly.

THE ICEBERG EFFECT

There is a difference between what the public perceive as their health care needs and their actual need, which is determined by health professionals. This is not entirely the fault of the patient but also due to a lack of effective

Table 28.1 National Statistics Socio-economic Classification (NS-SEC) of analytical classes

Class	Label
1	Managerial and professional occupations
2	Intermediate occupations
3	Small employers and own account workers
4	Lower supervisory and technical occupations
5	Semi-routine and routine occupations

SOCIOLOGY

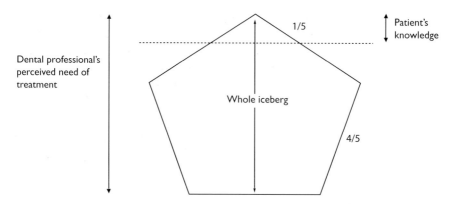

Figure 28.1 The iceberg effect (© Ruth McIntosh. Reproduced with permission)

communication by professionals – and is known in dentistry as the *iceberg effect* (Figure 28.1).

The dental professionals' perceived need of treatment is represented by the whole iceberg. The patient's knowledge of treatment required is represented by the tip of the iceberg.

The performance gap

Four fifths of the iceberg represents the *performance gap*. This is the difference between what professionals expect of patients and what patients think is needed. Health professionals may blame the patient for not acting on their advice, as they see patients as responsible for their own ill health. However, patients may be doing their best and are actually victims of their own personal/social circumstances. The *gap* can be reduced by education of both professionals and patients.

Victim blaming

What the patient sees as responsible action, the health professional (not understanding the circumstances) may see as irresponsibility. This is known as *victim blaming* and can lead to the breakdown of dental professional–patient relationships. The OHE can re-educate both sides, lessen the performance gap and preserve the relationship, as shown in the following example.

An example of how to lessen the performance gap

The problem:

The dentist suggests that a patient cleans around a bridge daily with a high-quality floss. The patient cannot afford this but is too embarrassed to tell the dentist. Therefore, the bridge is not regularly cleaned and dental problems occur. The dentist blames the patient for not acting on advice. The patient blames the dentist for not understanding their financial circumstances.

Negative result: the patient leaves the practice and goes elsewhere.

The solution:

Had an OHE been available when the bridge was fitted, the patient would have been more likely to reveal that the recommended floss was too expensive. The OHE could then:

- Find a compromise.

- Check out a cheaper alternative with the dentist (perhaps interdental bottle brushes, which unlike floss can be used more than once).

- Relay the information to the patient (who is happy with the less expensive compromise).

Positive result: the OHE will have negated the iceberg effect, closed the performance gap, prevented victim blaming and kept a patient for the practice.

Remember! Improved communication by health professionals may give a better understanding of patients' problems and difficulties and lead to an improved dental professional–patient relationship.

SELF-ASSESSMENT

1. Write short notes on socialisation, social classification, the iceberg effect and how health and social factors contribute to oral disease.

SOCIOLOGY

REFERENCES

1. Central Office of Information (2005) *Choosing Better Oral Health, An Oral Health Plan for England*. Department of Health, London.
2. Ireland, R. (2004) *Advanced Dental Nursing*, Blackwell Science Ltd., Oxford
3. National Statistics (May 2006) Available at www.statistics.gov.uk (Crown copyright material is reproduced with the permission of the Controller of HMSO).
4. Office for National Statistics (2000) *Adult Dental Health Survey (1998): Oral Health in the United Kingdom, 1998*. Stationery Office Books, London.

Chapter 29
Epidemiology

LEARNING OUTCOMES

By the end of this chapter you should be able to:

1. Define *epidemiology* and explain why it is useful in dentistry.

2. Name the UK organisation which collects and analyses epidemiological statistics.

3. State the years in which UK child and adult dental surveys are conducted and explain how the data collected is utilized.

4. List four terms frequently used in carrying out surveys.

5. Explain what an *index* is and how it is used in epidemiology. List two plaque indices; one oral hygiene index; one caries index and one periodontal index; a basic periodontal examination (BPE) index, and briefly summarise how they are used.

6. State the tasks which may be carried out in the mouth by the oral health educator (OHE).

WHAT IS EPIDEMIOLOGY?

Epidemiology is the study of the prevalence and distribution of disease within population groups[1]. It is concerned with studying the presence of disease in a community, country or region, and can help to ascertain the size, severity, spread and origin of a particular disease.

An *epidemiologist* deals with diseases in groups of people (whereas a clinician deals with disease in individuals). From epidemiology studies, decisions can be made on the allocation or targeting of resources throughout a community.

Epidemiology is the foundation upon which governments and local authorities plan preventive measures for future generations, such as the fluoridation of water and how many dentists will need to be trained in 20 or 30 years' time to meet demand.

The OHE needs to know a little about how surveys are used in epidemiology and how they are undertaken.

SURVEYS

Surveys are systems used to collect and record data vital to epidemiology and future planning.

Often, hundreds or thousands of subjects have to be surveyed, and the data must be recorded and analysed. Surveys must therefore be simple, reproducible and non-time-consuming.

The main UK government organisation concerned with collecting data is called the Office for National Statistics (ONS). As mentioned throughout this book, two of their surveys are of particular significance to the OHE:

- National survey of adult dental health 1998

- National survey of child dental health 2003

These two surveys are carried out every 10 years – adults in years ending with '8' and children in years ending with '3'. (An easy way to remember this is that children are smaller than adults and a '3' looks half the size of an '8'). Statistics are collected and recorded by community dental officers (often assisted by dental nurses), who examine sections of the population in their areas and chart results.

These statistics are sent to the ONS where they are analysed, collated and published in report form[2,3]. Reports can then be used by area authorities, considering for example, whether to fluoridate their water supply, or whether to implement procedures to control drinks sold in school tuck shops.

Survey terminology

The OHE must be familiar with four terms that are used in the context of epidemiological surveys:

1. *Screening* – refers to examining the population.

2. *Prevalence* – looks at how widespread a condition is in the population.

3. *Incidence* – how often a condition occurs.

4. *Distribution* – assesses where most disease occurs in the population.

INDICES

An *index* (plural *indices*) is a numerical method of measuring data used in a survey.

Before indices were devised, oral hygiene and the extent of disease were graded by terms such as *good*, *average* or *poor*. Obviously, this was

EPIDEMIOLOGY

unsatisfactory as one person's idea of *good* may differ from another. Factors such as the extent of plaque and calculus were not recorded.

It was not until the late 1940s that people began to work on reliable methods of measuring and grading data. In the 1960s and 1970s, indices (still in use now) were developed. Much of this work can be attributed to Scandinavians.

Examples of data that can be gathered using indices include:

- Extent of caries – how many in a population are affected?

- Extent of periodontal disease – how widespread is it?

- Oral hygiene – how effectively are people cleaning teeth?

- Presence of plaque (or debris) – which surfaces are most commonly missed?

- Tooth mobility – at what age do people often loose teeth from gum disease?

There are many indices (especially for plaque), although the OHE need only explore some of the simplest, which are used in conjunction with a disclosing solution to measure the extent of plaque on the teeth.

Silness and Löe plaque index (1964)[4]

The patient is disclosed and the presence of plaque noted as follows:

- Code 0 = No plaque deposits visible in the gingival area.

- Code 1 = Plaque deposits visible in the gingival area after disclosing.

Turesky plaque index (1970)

Many dental professionals are now using the Turesky index. This relatively simple method of measuring the presence of plaque, offers a high level of sensitivity and is a useful patient motivation tool.

Instructions for using Turesky index (P. Renton-Harper, personal communications):

1. Disclose the patient

2. Record buccal, labial, palatal, lingual surfaces for each tooth (using the index that follows)
   The Turesky index:

   0 = no plaque

   1 = Separate flecks of plaque at cervical tooth margin

2 = Thin, continuous band of plaque (up to 1 mm) at cervical margin

3 = Band of plaque more than 1 mm wide but covering less than $^1/_3$ of crown

4 = Plaque covering at least $^1/_3$ but less than $^2/_3$ of crown

5 = Plaque covering $^2/_3$ or more of crown

3. Calculate the percentage of plaque present:

$$\frac{\text{Total score (upper and lower arch)}}{\text{Divided by the number of teeth} \times 10} \times 100$$

Oral hygiene index (1960)[4]

The oral hygiene index (OHI) was developed by *Greene* and *Vermillion* and in its original form was a combination of two indices: a calculus index and a debris index for every tooth. They scored calculus as follows:

0 = None present

1 = Supragingival calculus covering less than $^1/_3$ of the tooth surface

2 = Supragingival calculus covering $^1/_3$ or $^2/_3$ of the tooth surface and small amounts of subgingival calculus present

3 = Supragingival calculus covering more than $^2/_3$ of tooth surface or continuous bands of subgingival calculus

The same scoring system was used for debris (plaque/food) and extrinsic staining. However, this index proved to be too complex and time consuming for general use, so Greene and Vermillion simplified it in 1964, facilitating its use in wider population groups. The resulting *simplified oral hygiene index* (OHI-S) selected only six tooth surfaces from different areas, as being representative of the whole mouth.

DMFT caries index (1930s)

The DMFT index (decayed, missing, filled teeth) is the most commonly used index in UK epidemiological surveys of caries. It was developed by Klein and Palmer in the 1930s and the fact that it is still in use today indicates its success[5]. An important point to remember with this index is that large-case letters (DMFT) denote permanent teeth, while small-case letters (dmft) denote deciduous teeth.

By counting the number of decayed, missing and filled teeth, it is possible to assess the extent of caries in a population. If the DMFT-S ($S = surfaces\ decayed\ or\ filled$) are counted, the technique becomes even more specific. (Scores of 1–5 are used.)

For example, a dentist and nurse survey a class of schoolchildren and record decayed, missing and filled teeth. For children a def(t) or def(s) index is used, where the 'e' stands for extracted deciduous teeth, rather than those which *are exfoliated* (fall out) naturally. A filled tooth scores 1. If they count the surfaces filled (e.g. a *three-surface filling*), the score for that tooth becomes 3. A tooth extracted because of caries scores 5 (five surfaces are missing).

Basic periodontal examination (BPE) index (1982)

The OHE need only be aware of one periodontal disease index. OHEs do not carry out this examination, but may assist the dentist or hygienist by recording the data.

This screening system is based on the Community Periodontal Index of Treatment Needs (CPITN), which was developed by the World Health Organisation (WHO) in 1982, and subsequently adapted by the British Society of Periodontology[6].

For periodontal examination, the dentition is divided into six sextants. The WHO probe is recommended when undertaking this examination. It has a ball end 0.5 mm in diameter, and a colour-coded area which extends from 3.5–5.5 mm and may also have a second colour-coded area running from 8.5–11.5 mm. Probing force should not exceed 20–25 g.

The probe tip is gently inserted into the gingival pocket and the depth of insertion read against the colour coding. The total extent of the pocket should be explored, by 'walking' the probe around the pocket. At least six points on each tooth should be examined: mesiobuccal, midbuccal, distobuccal, distopalatal, midpalatal and mesiopalatal (or lingual on lowers).

For each sextant, the highest score together with a '*' symbol, if appropriate, is recorded (Code * denotes furcation involvement or if there is loss of attachment of 7 mm or more). A sextant with only one tooth is recorded as missing

Table 29.1 Example of possible highest scores in sextants

Right premolars and molars	Central incisors and canines	Left premolars and molars
Upper right (UR) 4–7 Code 3	Upper 3–3 Code 1	Upper left (UL) 4–7 Code 3
Lower right (LR) 4–7 Code 4	Lower 3–3 Code 2	Lower left (LL) 4–7 Code 3

(+) and the score is included in the adjacent sextant. A simple box is used to record the scores for each sextant.

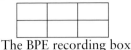

The BPE recording box

The following codes are used for diagnosis and treatment needs:

Code 0: Pockets 0–3 mm. Healthy gingivae with no bleeding on probing.

Treatment: no treatment required.

Code 1: Pockets 0–3.5 mm. Coloured area of probe remains completely visible in the deepest pocket in the sextant. No calculus or defective margins are detected. There is bleeding after probing.

Treatment: oral hygiene instruction (OHI).

Code 2: Pockets 0–3.5 mm. Coloured area of probe remains completely visible in the deepest pocket in the sextant. Supra- or subgingival calculus is detected or the defective margin of a filling or crown.

Treatment: OHI plus removal of calculus and correction of plaque retentive margins of fillings or crowns.

Patients whose codes are 0, 1 and 2 should be screened again at intervals of 1 year.

Code 3: Pockets 3.5–5.5 mm. Coloured area of probe remains partially visible in the deepest pocket of the sextant.

Treatment: as code 2, but a longer time will be required for treatment. Plaque and bleeding scores should be recorded at the start of treatment and when the patient returns for an assessment visit after treatment is completed – usually 3 months.

Code 4: Pockets 5.5 mm and above. Coloured area of probe disappears into the pocket indicating probing depths of at least 6 mm.

Treatment: a full probing depth chart is required together with bleeding and plaque indices, recession and furcation involvement. Together with any other relevant clinical details. Individual intra-oral radiographs for teeth with loss of attachment greater than 7 mm or furcation involvement.

Patients with 'code 4 and/or *' should undergo a course of periodontal treatment including oral hygiene instruction, root surface debridement and/or local or systemic antibiotic therapy as needed. This should be carried out by a suitably qualified person, such as a dental hygienist, a periodontist or a dental practitioner with relevant experience.

Patients who have undergone a course of periodontal therapy should have full mouth charting repeated after a minimum of 3 months.

Remember! The names and dates of these indices.

Remember! An OHE can use plaque and bleeding indices in education sessions to motivate patients and evaluate teaching and may disclose patients (with the patient's and dentist's permission). They may also demonstrate brushing in the mouth, but must not clean the teeth or use instruments (e.g. a pocket probe), as this constitutes the *practice of dentistry*.

SELF-ASSESSMENT

1. Define epidemiology and describe its purpose.

2. What name is given to methods used to collect and record data, and what is this data used for?

3. Name the UK body which collects and analyses statistics.

4. Name two surveys (including dates) of particular interest to the OHE and describe an easy way to remember the dates of UK dental surveys.

5. What is an index and why are indices used when carrying out surveys?

6. Name two indices used to measure oral hygiene (i.e. calculus and debris present and the presence of plaque).

7. Name the index most commonly used to measure caries incidence (stating how to differentiate between permanent and deciduous teeth).

8. What does BPE stand for and what treatment would be appropriate for a patient with code 4?

9. In one sentence for each, define screening, prevalence, incidence and distribution.

10. Write a brief paragraph describing what tasks an OHE may or may not carry out in the patient's mouth.

REFERENCES

1. National Examining Board for Dental Nurses (2001) *Course Syllabus: Certificate in Oral Health Education*, NEBDN, Fleetwood, Lancashire.
2. Office for National Statistics (2000) *Adult Dental Health Survey (1998): Oral Health in the United Kingdom, 1998.* Stationery Office Books, London.

3. Office for National Statistics (2004) *2003 Dental Health Survey of Children and Young People*. Stationery Office Books, London.
4. Collins, W.J., Walsh, T., Figures, K. (1999) *A Handbook for Dental Hygienists*, 4th edn. Butterworth Heinemann, Oxford.
5. Fejerskov, O., Kidd, E. (2004) *Dental Caries, The Disease and Its Clinical Management*, Blackwell Munksgaard, Oxford.
6. World Health Organisation (2002) Technical assessment of WHO – 621, periodontal probe made in Brazil, *Brazilian Dental Journal*, 13(1), 61–65.

EPIDEMIOLOGY

Chapter 30
Evidence-based prevention

LEARNING OUTCOMES

By the end of this chapter you should be able to:

1. Explain the meaning of the term *evidence-based prevention*.
2. Explain (giving examples) what is meant by primary, secondary and tertiary dental health prevention.
3. State the recommendations of the National Institute for Clinical Excellence (NICE) report on the frequency of dental attendance.

PREVENTION IS BETTER THAN CURE

The importance of *prevention*, which UK OHEs have been teaching for many years, is now recognised by the UK Department of Health (and implemented through government initiatives), as vital in improving the general and dental health of the nation[1]. In 2002, the NHS identified *prevention* as playing a key role in combating dental disease[2].

Prevention encompasses a wide range of strategies designed to prevent the development of dental disease and should be initiated in early childhood.

Examples of prevention include:

- Fluoridation of drinking water.
- Administration of topical fluoride in toothpaste and by other means if thought necessary (i.e. tablets and drops for infants, mouthwash, gels and varnish for older children and adults).
- Fissure sealing first permanent molars.
- Choosing a diet low in extrinsic sugars.
- Effective toothbrushing and mouth cleaning.

- Regular dental check-ups – that screen for oral cancer as well as caries and periodontal disease in older people.

Evidence-based prevention

In the UK, much emphasis is now placed on the importance of *evidence-based prevention* by the dental profession, the General Dental Council and the government. The term is used when research has shown that a particular strategy in reducing dental disease has been effective. For example: it can be scientifically proved that the addition of fluoride to drinking water and toothpaste reduces caries. This is evidence-based prevention.

If, however, there is no tangible proof that a particular oral health strategy, such as reducing dietary sugars, has reduced the caries rate, then although it is to be recommended, it cannot be said to be evidence-based. The OHE can stress the importance of less sugar in the diet, but there is no way of making patients carry out this advice. This does not mean that such non-evidence-based advice is wrong and should not be given.

Scientific evidence to support advice given to patients can be found on the Cochrane Network[3] – a series of reviews of scientific evidence initiated by Professor Archie Cochrane in the 1970s. Cochrane saw the need to establish an international network of groups which would simplify evidence-based decision-making in clinical practice.

Several organisations have been set up with the aim of standardising and integrating the methods used to develop guidelines for clinical practice. One of these is the Scottish International Guidelines Network (SIGN).

Primary dental health prevention

Primary dental health prevention is directed at healthy patients and aims to prevent illness and improve the quality of health and life. Examples of primary dental health prevention include:

- Fluoridation of drinking water.

- Advice to pregnant mothers and parents of small children on avoiding or reducing unnecessary sugars, and stressing the importance of brushing regularly with fluoride paste.

- Fissure sealing – from second molars to first permanent molars before decay can develop.

- Advice to pre-teenage children on the dangers to the oral cavity of smoking and drinking alcohol.

Secondary dental health prevention

Secondary dental health prevention is directed at patients with an existing condition, whose full health could be restored by taking appropriate action, or whose disease can be prevented from further progression. *At risk* patients are an important target group for secondary dental health prevention. Examples of secondary dental health prevention include helping patients towards:

- Resolution of gingivitis (particularly in the young). Simple oral health measures are applied, before progression to periodontitis.

- Remineralisation of early caries by using a fluoride toothpaste and modifying diet.

- Bringing children to the dentist for fillings whilst cavities are still small.

- Control of dental manifestations of systemic disease (e.g. diabetes).

Tertiary dental health prevention

Tertiary dental health prevention is directed at people who have a terminal or unresolvable condition or disability. It is aimed at educating the patient to make the most of the remaining potential for healthy living and where possible avoid unnecessary hardships, restrictions and complications. Relatives and carers of patients in '*at risk*' groups may also need help and advice. Examples of tertiary dental health care include:

- Care of a crown or bridge.

- Care of partial or full dentures.

- Maintaining oral health when advanced periodontal disease is present.

- Care of the mouth when the patient has a medical condition that makes effective oral hygiene difficult.

Another important aspect of prevention is the routine check-up carried out by the dentist. UK dentists have been given guidelines by NICE, which was established to determine evidence-based guidelines in the NHS. However, many dental surgeons prefer to stick to six-monthly check-ups for adults and more frequent checks for children.

Recommendations of the NICE report

In 2004, NICE produced a guide on how often dentists should carry out routine check-ups. Much scientific literature was reviewed in order to assess risks to patients if dental check-ups (six-monthly) were carried out less frequently. The

EVIDENCE-BASED PREVENTION

findings published in a report in 2003 are as follows[4]:

1. There is little need for six-monthly check-ups over any other frequency of recall.

2. Shortening the interval to less than 6 months results in small reductions in caries, but not other conditions.

3. Changes are determined by individual risk (patients' needs may vary).

4. Making the interval between check-ups longer than 6 months is more cost-effective.

NICE also suggested that reviews for patients on the basis of disease risk assessments should be undertaken. Reviews could be undertaken between:

- 3 and 24 months (for adults)
- 3 and 12 months (for children)

The dental professional (usually the dentist), has the responsibility to use their clinical judgement when determining the interval between check-ups, but should consult the patient or carer when making the decision.

SELF-ASSESSMENT

1. Write notes on what is meant by the term *evidence-based prevention*, and describe the role of the OHE in primary health care.

2. Give examples of secondary and tertiary prevention in relation to oral health.

3. List the recommendations of the NICE report.

REFERENCES

1. Department of Health (2005) *Choosing Better Oral Health: An Oral Health Plan for England*. Department of Health Publications, London.
2. Department of Health (2002) *NHS Dentistry: Options for Change*. Department of Health Publications, London.
3. Cochrane Network (May 2006) Available at www.cochrane.org.
4. Steele, J. (2006) *The NICE Guidelines on Patient Recall: Common Sense or Compulsion?* In *Action in Practice, Wrigley Oral Healthcare in Action*, Vol. 8, Issue 3.

EVIDENCE-BASED PREVENTION

Chapter 31
UK dental services

LEARNING OUTCOMES

By the end of this chapter you should be able to:

1. Briefly explain the establishment of the UK National Health Service (NHS) and give reasons why little NHS dental treatment is now available.

2. Describe the ways in which the public can obtain dental treatment.

3. State the organisation responsible for regulations concerning all members of the dental team.

4. Show awareness of ongoing changes in the provision of NHS services and the implications of these changes for patients and dentists.

5. Explain what is meant by *clinical governance*, with reference to the *Donabedian concept*.

GENERAL DENTAL SERVICE

The NHS was set up in 1948 with the aim of providing free medical and dental care for the whole population, regardless of social status. Funded by the government from taxation, it soon became the envy of the world.

Over the years, there have inevitably been many changes to the NHS, including the provision of dental care. Perhaps the most significant change is that adults have had to pay increasing amounts towards the costs of NHS dental treatment. However, pregnant/nursing mothers, children in full-time education and those receiving certain benefits and allowances are entitled to free dental treatment.

HISTORY OF PRIVATE DENTAL PRACTICES

In 1990, the government made radical changes to the way NHS dentists were paid and as a result many dentists left the NHS and adopted private schemes. Often such schemes are not liked by patients, but seen as inevitable. Many private practices still continue to provide free treatment for *exempt groups*, but cost is still a major factor in discouraging certain population groups from attending. The current government (at the time of writing) is attempting to remedy this situation in a number of ways using *primary care trusts* (PCTs), and financial incentives.

Primary care trusts

PCTs have been set up countrywide and are responsible for the implementation of new contractual arrangements for NHS dentistry. Their oral health remit is to:

- Ensure that improving oral health is an integral part of their *local delivery plans*.
- Liaise with local authorities to ensure that improving oral health is included in joint planning objectives.
- Ensure that dental services they commission have an evidence-based preventive focus.
- Ensure that they are able to obtain appropriate 'health need' information and advice when developing local programmes.
- Consider whether water fluoridation is appropriate locally.

Financial incentives

The government has offered financial incentives to dentists who remain within the NHS.

New terminology introduced in 2006 refers to treatment as *Units of Dental Activity*. Dentists carrying out NHS work are required to complete a designated amount of units. If targets are not achieved, they are required to accept other NHS patients referred to by PCTs.

Emergency 'out of hours' services are run by PCTs, using access centres, A&E hospital departments and emergency slots with GDPs.

UK DENTAL SERVICES

COMMUNITY DENTAL SERVICE (CDS)

Some dental personnel are employed by NHS Trusts and work within the community, which covers hospitals, clinics and health centres, treating patients with special needs, those with phobias, pregnant mothers and children in low social groups. Community dental officers treat people in their own homes, and in residential and nursing homes (known as domiciliary care) if they are unable to attend a surgery. Some officers visit schools to carry out dental screenings for the purposes of collecting data, which is used for planning future services (dental screening of schoolchildren is not considered a dental examination).

Many parents do not take their children to the dentist because they misconstrue these epidemiological screenings as check-ups. The OHE should ensure that parents or carers are aware that they do need to register children with a dentist. PCTs use funding from the government to purchase all medical and dental services for their areas.

Many CDSs are now incorporated with personal dental services (PDS). However, it is currently confusing as to exactly how this will be organised and it is envisaged that the scheme may operate differently in various parts of the country.

Some PCTs cover *special care* and PDS for people who are unable to register with an NHS practice. After one course of treatment, patients are told they must find their own GDP, which at the current time, is very difficult. Indeed, many patients have been forced to adopt an 'only go when I have a problem with my teeth' attitude, and end up returning to the PDS (usually in pain). This is not acceptable to patients or dentists and goes against the idea of preventive dental care. The care delivered by the PDS acts as a safety net. The role of an OHE in delivering information on self-help skills and holding awareness-raising sessions (for unregistered people especially) is extremely important.

HOSPITAL DENTAL SERVICE

In university dental hospitals, patients are treated by students as part of their training (supervised by qualified personnel). GDPs can refer patients to specialised clinics within hospitals for diagnosis and treatment of oral diseases that are not treatable in general practice, but there are often long waiting lists for anything but emergencies.

Cases treated include advanced periodontal disease, oral cancer, orthodontics and other needs such as maxillofacial trauma and facial deformity (e.g. cleft lip and/or palate – usually picked up through the hospital service after birth).

UK DENTAL SERVICES

REGULATIONS GOVERNING DENTISTRY

The General Dental Council (GDC), a body made up of dentists, other health professionals and lay members, sets the regulations by which all dental professionals (including dental nurses) known as dental care professionals (DCPs) are governed. The law has recently been revised to allow professionals to carry out procedures for which they are trained and in which they have demonstrated competence[1].

Dental nurses must not carry out procedures in the oral cavity that constitute the *practice of dentistry*. This is a *grey area*, but is generally taken to mean that no dental instrument should be used by a dental nurse within the mouth. OHEs are advised to seek permission from their employer and the patient before demonstrating toothbrushing/flossing and other procedures within the mouth.

If dentists are uncertain about what procedures a nurse may carry out, they should seek advice from their dental indemnity company. With *registration*, nurses are required to provide their own indemnity and can therefore consult their own company if asked to carry out procedures for patients that they are not happy about.

The NEBDN Certificate in oral health education gives nurses the competency to carry out oral health education unsupervised to patients (under direction from the dentist). However, the dentist is ultimately responsible for any work carried out by members of staff, including dental nurses.

Clinical governance

Avedis Donabedian, Professor of Public Health in Michigan, USA, developed a concept of measuring the quality of health care given to patients by professionals in 1969 and is regarded by many professionals worldwide as having transformed the way health care is delivered.

Donabedian's concept was one of the theories which led to clinical governance and quality control in dental practices and trusts; requirements for staff to have appropriate and recognised qualifications, continuing professional development (CPD), and practice inspections to ensure that equipment is up to date and conforms to health and safety regulations[2].

Clinical governance was introduced to the NHS in 1998 and was designed to bring a systematic approach to the delivery of high-quality health care. Private practices are also required to comply with the requirements of quality control.

The *Donabedian concept* is based on three principles[3]:

- Structure

- Process

- Outcome

UK DENTAL SERVICES

These principles, when applied to providing quality dental care, can be explained as:

- Structure – provision of facilities (e.g. surgery access, provision for the disabled, modern equipment); and organisation of the practice: staff training, qualifications and CPD, patient–staff ratio and varied attributes of the personnel (special qualities they bring to the practice to help patients).

- Process – what the dentist and team do in the delivery of care to the patients, from taking and regularly updating medical histories to the technical process of delivering excellent treatment. Attention to health and safety of patients and staff at all times.

- Outcome – producing evidence that shows that patients are satisfied with the quality of care (e.g. via short questionnaires, when they return for routine checkups); offering to redo any treatment which has fallen short of patients' expectations free of charge; developing good relationships with patients so that they feel they can complain if not satisfied, and that complaints or suggestions will be promptly followed-up.

SELF-ASSESSMENT

1. When was the NHS established and how is it funded?
2. What led to many dentists leaving the NHS and practising independently or privately?
3. Briefly explain the various ways in which the public can obtain dental treatment.
4. Describe the changes to NHS treatment implemented in 2006.
5. Name the body responsible for regulations concerning dental nurses and the dental team.
6. What should a dental nurse do if asked to demonstrate oral health procedures in a patient's mouth?
7. Briefly explain what is meant by clinical governance, with reference to the Donabedian concept.

UK DENTAL SERVICES

REFERENCES

1. General Dental Council (2005) *Standards for Dental Professionals*. General Dental Council, London.
2. Rattan, R. (2007) Quality in healthcare: what does it mean? *Smile Journal*, 3(2), 18–19.
3. Kovner, C.T. (1989) Nurse–patient agreement and outcomes after surgery, *Western Journal of Nursing Research*, 11(1), 7–19.

Chapter 32

Oral health promotion

LEARNING OUTCOMES

By the end of this chapter you should be able to:

1. Distinguish between oral health promotion and oral health education.
2. Briefly explain the Ottawa Charter.
3. Explain why oral health promotion and education are not always effective.

WHAT IS ORAL HEALTH PROMOTION?

It is easy to confuse the terms oral health education and oral health promotion, and it is important for oral health educators (OHEs) to know the difference between them and where the two areas overlap. Oral health education is part of the wider aspect of oral health promotion which involves local, national and even international cooperation. 'Oral health promotion attempts to make the healthier choices the easier choices'[1]. It is about making wider changes, which will enable people to make healthier choices.

THE OTTAWA CHARTER

In 1986, WHO produced a document called *The Ottawa Charter*, which set out strategies for effective health promotion, including[2]:

- Building healthy public policy (e.g. legislation exempting toothpaste from VAT, adding fluoride to water).
- Local authority healthy eating policies.
- Creating supported environments (putting policies into action by making the healthy choices easy).

- Developing individual knowledge and skills in those who deal with the public, including doctors, dental personnel, pharmacists, caterers, teachers and nursery staff.

- Supporting community action – working with voluntary groups in communities to care for the health in their particular community.

- Re-orientating health services towards prevention and ensuring that all health professionals give the same message.

Twenty years on, the UK government published *Choosing Better Oral Health*, which was delivered to all NHS dental practices by the Department of Health in 2006[3]. It sets out, in considerable detail, the key steps which can be taken to improve oral health. It is recommended that all OHE students familiarise themselves with this document.

DEFINING PEOPLE'S NEEDS

If oral health promotion is to be effective, it is recognised that the Ottawa Charter needs to be implemented (for authorities, organisations, groups and individuals), continually revised, and delivered to the public in acceptable ways. In order to do this, it is necessary to define people's 'needs' (rather than 'wants'). For example: the population *needs* fluoridated water, the British Dental Association recommends it, the House of Lords have endorsed it, but large groups within communities still object to it, so that it cannot be implemented.

Epidemiological surveys[4] show that people in poorer, deprived areas suffer far greater dental disease than those in more prosperous areas and the needs expressed by people in poorer areas are more likely to be free treatment, rather than water fluoridation. This is known as *felt need*, and should be taken into account when professionals are assessing what they call *normative need* (the measures that they know will improve oral health).

The overall aim of oral health promotion is to influence the social norms of a community towards change and improvement (e.g. water fluoridation, smoking cessation). Greatest benefit will ultimately be obtained by combining *high-risk approaches* (where groups or individuals thought to be at highest risk of disease are targeted), with the *population approach* (such as water fluoridation).

WHY DOES INCREASING KNOWLEDGE NOT CHANGE BEHAVIOUR?

In recent years, there has been a radical change in the concept of health education as a whole. It used to be thought that providing people with the facts to

ORAL HEALTH PROMOTION

change to a healthy lifestyle was sufficient (as the dental profession in general and OHEs in particular try to do), but it is now recognised that this does not always work.

So why do people not change their behaviours when they are told about the risks to their general and dental health from practices (e.g. smoking and eating a high-sugar diet)? The reasons are complex and involve many factors, including:

- Community reasons (e.g. water not fluoridated).
- Social factors (conforming to social norms).
- Economic reasons – sweets still seen as a relatively cheap expression of love.
- Lack of knowledge-skills – people cannot change their behaviour unless they have the education and knowledge to do so.
- Some population groups do not visit dental professionals regularly, or ever.

However, the most recent surveys of adult dental health (1998)[4] and child dental health (2003)[5] in the UK show that the overall health of the nation is better than it has ever been, although there are still regional and cultural variations and much to be achieved.

Fifty years ago, most adults expected to lose many, if not all, of their teeth in middle age (40–60 years). This was the norm and was due to a number of reasons:

- They, like their parents, were frightened of dentists and believed tales that dental procedures were painful.
- In the years following the Second World War, jobs were difficult to obtain and money short. Parents had not been able to afford dental treatment and it was some time after the introduction of the NHS that people realised that they could access dental treatment free or inexpensively.
- Treatment of extensive caries took priority after the war years and many people lost teeth due to unrecognised or undiagnosed periodontal disease.
- Sweets came off ration in the early 1950s and the harm they did to children's teeth was not fully recognised for some years. Children often had baby teeth extracted and it was not recognised that early loss of deciduous teeth caused orthodontic problems later in childhood.
- Some social groups regarded it as a kindness to provide a 'dowry' for daughters about to get married by arranging for all their teeth to be extracted and dentures provided.
- Dental treatment was aimed at cure rather than prevention until comparatively recently.

ORAL HEALTH PROMOTION

Now, early in the twenty-first century, dental professionals commonly see patients in their seventies, eighties and even nineties who still have many of their natural teeth, and increasing numbers of caries-free teenagers and young adults. This is largely due to improvements in general health; higher income in many population groups; attention to healthier diets; fluoride in toothpaste; improvements in dental treatment, and the influence of the media.

This improvement in health can also be attributed to education and this is where OHEs come in – by improving the dental health of the nation's individuals. OHEs should never underestimate their abilities to work in education and promotion together with other professionals, keep abreast of current developments in dentistry, and put forward suggestions to improve patients' health and lives.

The *Giant of Dentistry* has arisen from a long slumber and is moving forward at a rapid pace. With government, national, local and community organisations working together with an army of well-trained, enthusiastic OHEs and promoters, tooth loss could well become a thing of the past.

SELF-ASSESSMENT

1. Define and differentiate between oral health promotion and education.

2. Briefly explain the Ottawa Charter.

3. Write short notes on why oral health education does not always work, including reference to the changes in the way dental care professionals are approaching education and promotion.

REFERENCES

1. Blinkhorn, A.S. (2001) *Notes on Oral Health*, 5th edn. Eden Bianchi Press, Manchester.
2. Ireland, R. (2004) *Advanced Dental Nursing*, Blackwell Science Ltd., Oxford.
3. Department of Health (2005) *Choosing Better Oral Health: An Oral Health Plan for England*. Department of Health Publications, London.
4. Office for National Statistics (2000) *Adult Dental Health Survey (1998): Oral Health in the United Kingdom, 1998*. Stationery Office Books, London.
5. Office for National Statistics (2004) *2003 Dental Health Survey of Children and Young People*. Stationery Office Books, London.

ORAL HEALTH PROMOTION

Index